PREVEN

CW01558879

ALZHEIMᴇʀ ᴐ

ALZHEIMER'S FACTORS, PREVENTION STEPS AND FOODS THAT PREVENT OR SLOW ALZHEIMER'S, RECIPES FOR ALZHEIMER'S PREVENTION DIET

JOSEPH VEEBE

Books in this Series:

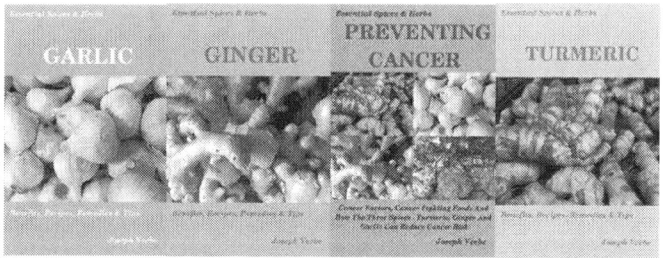

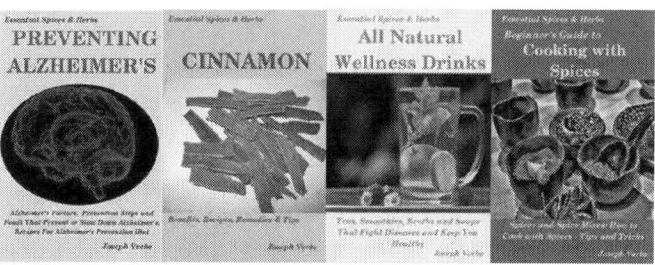

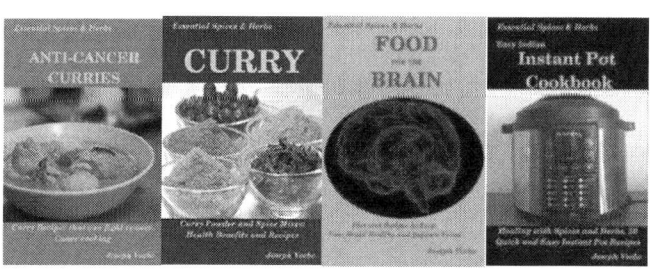

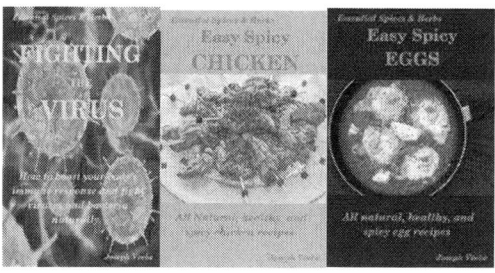

WHY I WROTE THIS BOOK

Many of us have heard that spices and herbs are good for our health, but we hardly incorporate these into western cuisine. Even though there has been more awareness lately on the health benefits of herbs/spices as part of natural alternatives or supplements to medicines, very few regularly incorporate spices and herbs in their diet. Some people hit nutritional stores to get natural supplements. While supplements are good, getting the same through natural foods is definitely preferable and can offer many nutrients that are simply not available in supplements.

Lately, more and more studies have been conducted on the health benefits of spices, herbs, and other natural, unprocessed foods. These studies have shown that natural foods, herbs, and spices are effective in preventing and treating many modern debilitating diseases such as cancer, heart diseases, and Alzheimer's.

Researchers estimate that about one-third of all Alzheimer's cases are preventable or at least delayed by proper lifestyle changes. As the population ages, the risk of Alzheimer's increases significantly. While there are no cures for dementia and Alzheimer's at the moment, there are several ways to prevent, slow down progress or delay the onset of Alzheimer's disease. This book details various ways, including diet, that help in preventing or delaying Alzheimer's. Alzheimer's factors are discussed, and several prevention steps are identified. The focus of this book is prevention by food and diet. I have listed many brain-boosting foods that include superfoods, spices, and herbs that have shown through evidence to benefit maintaining a healthy brain. By combining all three ingredients in cooking, many dishes become brain foods that help in the fight against the dreadful Alzheimer's disease.

TABLE OF CONTENTS

CHAPTER 1. INTRODUCTION

INTRODUCTION

Alzheimer's disease is the most common form of dementia, a progressive, irreversible brain disorder. The effect of Alzheimer's is that brain functions such as memory, cognition, focus, and rational thinking are all impaired and worsen over time. The nerve cells in the brain degenerate or die, the brain shrinks, and all daily functions become increasingly difficult. Alzheimer's disease is fatal.

Worldwide, approximately 50 million people live with Alzheimer's or other forms of dementia. Developed or western countries are the most affected. The most affected countries are Finland, the US, Canada, Iceland, Sweden, Switzerland, Norway, Denmark, Netherlands, Belgium, Spain, Australia, France, and the UK in that order. The Mediterranean and South Asian countries are among the least affected. Countries with the lowest Alzheimer's rate include India, Georgia, Cambodia, Tajikistan, Kyrgyzstan, Uzbekistan, and Singapore.

The ratio between death rate due to Alzheimer's in western countries to that of the lowest rate countries are several orders of magnitude. For example, the US has 100 (45 incidents in 100, 000) times the Alzheimer's death rate compared to India (0.46 in 100,000). This is indeed very worrisome, and Alzheimer's could hit epidemic proportions in the US and other western countries by 2050.

Facts about Alzheimer's disease in the US:

- In 2017, about 5.5 million people were living with Alzheimer's disease.

- Of the 5.5 million, 5.3 million were age 65 and older and about 200,000 were early onset incidents (Alzheimer's incident at younger than 65 years).

- About 5% of Alzheimer's incidents are due to genetic factors.

- 1 in 10 people over 65 years have Alzheimer's.

- The risk for Alzheimer's doubles every 5 years after the age of 65.

- After the age of 85, 1 in 2 people have some form of Alzheimer's dementia.

- 2 out of 3 Alzheimer's patients are women.

- About 750,000 deaths were attributed to Alzheimer's in 2017.

- In 2015, the estimated cost of Alzheimer's for the US was about $226 billion. It is expected to cross a trillion by the year 2050.

- Medicaid cost alone is an estimated 44 billion in 2017.

- As the baby boomers age, the number of Alzheimer's cases is expected to more than double by 2050 from current levels.

While significant research is being conducted into Alzheimer's disease, researchers are yet to find the cause of Alzheimer's. Researchers have identified changes the brain undergoes during Alzheimer's through various imaging techniques.

Researchers are working to identify the causes of the changes in the brain during Alzheimer's. At the same time, the pharmaceutical industry has been working on various potential treatments, some for symptoms, some for coping with the disease, and some clinical trials for treatments. Many of the trials for these experimental drugs have failed. The hope is that soon scientists will be able to definitely identify the cause and that will lead to an effective treatment.

Given the state of treatment, and the huge impact on the patients, caregivers, and the economy, one should give serious consideration to ways for preventing, delaying the onset of or if possible, slowing down or reversing Alzheimer's progression. Delaying Alzheimer's even by a couple of years has huge benefits for patients and their families both in quality of life and in finances. This book is all about preventing Alzheimer's.

After reading and reviewing much information and data about Alzheimer's, this author believes that lifestyle is the most significant factor in Alzheimer's incidents. How can one explain nearly 100 times Alzheimer's rate in Western countries compared to much less developed countries such as India, and some of the other Asian and African countries? Of course, there is a higher life expectancy in the western world that can account partly for the higher Alzheimer's rate. But it is hard to explain 100 times Alzheimer's incidents in the US compared to India. This author considers the following key factors leading to the low level of Alzheimer's in the 3rd world. 1) Food habits – there is virtually no fast food, less processed food, less meat, and more freshly prepared food often using medicinal spices and herbs and consumed in moderation.2) There are significantly more family and social ties and engagements (not the Facebook or twitter kind but real family and community engagements), 3) less stress, 4) less exposure to chemicals, heavy metals, and other harmful substances, and 5) less automation and other modern-day conveniences, which helps people end up doing more mental and physical exercise as part of their everyday routines, 6) less intake of prescription drugs. This book tries to address each of these factors while giving particular attention to food and what we put into our bodies.

CHAPTER 2. UNDERSTANDING DEMENTIA AND ALZHEIMER'S

Alzheimer's is one of those debilitating neurological conditions that we all dread. The risk of getting Alzheimer's grows with age.

As per www.alz.org, Alzheimer's disease is a progressive brain disorder that damages and eventually destroys brain cells, leading to memory loss and changes in thinking and other brain functions.

While the human body's capabilities, including brain function, deteriorate as we age, significant brain damage to cause Alzheimer's or other dementia happens at old age. When Alzheimer's is diagnosed at the middle age or before the age of 65, it is usually considered to be early-onset Alzheimer's. About 5% of all Alzheimer's cases are in the early-onset category.

While the rate of progressive decline in brain function is slow at the onset, it gets worse with time and age. Brain function decline accelerates, and brain cells eventually die over time. Currently, there is no cure for Alzheimer's.

DEMENTIA

In simple terms, dementia is a condition where a person's ability to do normal everyday functions are impacted by forgetfulness. Alzheimer's is the most common form of dementia. About 60-80 percent of dementia cases fall under the heading of Alzheimer's.

BRAIN CHANGES IN ALZHEIMER'S PATIENTS

There have been numerous researches into understanding Alzheimer's – causes, the changes in the brain over the course of Alzheimer's disease, and also prevention and cure.

During the course of Alzheimer's disease progression, the brain undergoes a number of changes:

1. The overall brain size shrinks because of Alzheimer's disease. This is due to brain cell death and tissue loss throughout the brain. Over time, the shrinkage could be very dramatic.

2. The cortex shrivels up and as a result of the area of the brain involved in thinking, planning, and remembering, is damaged. The hippocampus area of the cortex shrinks significantly and as a result, formations of new memories are severely impacted.

3. Alzheimer's brain tissues have fewer nerve cells and synapses than a healthy brain. **Plaques**, clusters of protein fragments built up between nerve cells, are formed, which impact the transmittal of the brain signals that form memories, feelings, and thoughts. These plaques are essentially formed by the **beta-amyloid** protein pieces sticking together and blocking brain signals.

4. Another protein called **tau** which typically forms the tracks or pathway for essential nutrients (the brain food) gets tangled up. As the tau protein forms **tangles** (twisted strands), the brain food (nutrients and other essential supplies) do not have a proper track or pathway for moving through the cells and nourishing them. As a result, cells start to die.

5. Due to the plaques and tangles in the brain, the connection (synapses) among brain cells responsible for memory, communication, and learning are impacted. And over time these plaques and tangles start to grow, and the brain's abilities are progressively impacted.

6. With the brain cells under attack, the body triggers its immune system and causes inflammation in the brain which worsens the disease.

STAGES OF ALZHEIMER'S

The rate of progression in Alzheimer's varies significantly between patients depending on a number of factors, including lifestyle, food, genetics, and others.

Early Alzheimer's

In early Alzheimer's the brain changes may begin way before it is diagnosed. In some cases, brain changes may start 20-25 years before diagnosis. In this stage, beta-amyloid plaques and tau tangles start to form. Current tests are inadequate to detect this stage of Alzheimer's.

Mild to moderate Alzheimer's

Mild to moderate Alzheimer's generally lasts from 2-10 years before it becomes severe. In this stage, the brain develops more plaques and tangles that start to impact memory, thinking, and planning capabilities. As a result, work or social life starts getting impacted. Individuals have trouble remembering names, expressing thoughts, or planning their day to day lives. Most often, these troubles help in the diagnosis of Alzheimer's condition. In this stage, individuals may easily get confused, speaking and understanding can get difficult as the condition progresses, there could be changes in personality and behavior and they can have trouble recognizing family and friends.

Severe Alzheimer's

Severe Alzheimer's stage may last from 1-5 years. This stage is the most severe condition where the individuals become incapable of caring for themselves. They lose the ability to communicate and do not recognize family and loved ones. In this stage, there is significant brain cell death and overall brain shrinkage.

SYMPTOMS OF ALZHEIMER'S

As discussed above, the most common symptom is difficulty in learning and remembering new information. This is because, during the early stages, the part that helps in learning and processing new information is the one that gets affected most. As the disease progresses, many other symptoms appear such as remembering past events, time and place, names of friends and family, and other details. Behavioral changes, mood swings, disorientation, difficulty in speaking, swallowing, and walking. Caring for themselves becomes increasingly difficult.

CAUSES AND RISK FACTORS

The researchers are not clear on the actual cause of Alzheimer's disease. However, they know many factors that can trigger the disease. Scientists believe that Alzheimer's is the result of several factors coming together. The biggest risk factors are old age, genetics, and a family history of Alzheimer's.

Age

The risk of Alzheimer's increases with age. After the age of 65, the risk for Alzheimer's doubles every 5 years and after the age of 85, the risk is about 50 percent.

Family History

Research has shown that family history plays a part in Alzheimer's risk. Those who have someone in their immediate family with Alzheimer's are at a greater risk than those without any family members having Alzheimer's. The risk increases based on the number of immediate family members with Alzheimer's.

Genetics

The twenty-three human chromosome pairs contain more than 30,000 genes that code the genetic blueprint for a human being. Out of these, 4 gene mutations or variations are identified (as of yet) to cause or impact the risk of developing Alzheimer's. Three out of these 4 are inherited genes. They are Amyloid precursor protein (APP), Presenilin- 1 (PS-1), and Presenilin- 2 (PS-2). These three inherited genes with mutations can cause Alzheimer's. Please note that genes causing "familial Alzheimer's" are very rare and account for less than 5 percent of Alzheimer's cases worldwide.

The fourth gene, Apolipoprotein E-e4 (APOE4) is considered a risk gene. This gene has the greatest impact on the risk of Alzheimer's. While this gene is the greatest risk, having this mutation does not mean the person will develop Alzheimer's.

Lifestyle

While there is no conclusive evidence of certain lifestyle impacts Alzheimer's, it evident that unhealthy eating including processed foods, foods that cause inflammation, or cardiovascular issues can impact brain health as well. A diet that is high in anti-oxidants, anti-inflammatory compounds and that helps boost immunity such DASH or Mediterranean diet is good for overall health and potentially slow down or delay Alzheimer's, if not outrightly prevent it. Besides diet, common taking common prescription medication (anticholinergic drugs) can increase the risk of dementia as much as 50% as found out in a recent (2019) study.

Early Detection

As there is no cure for Alzheimer's to date, the focus has been on 1) early detection so treatment can begin before irreversible brain damage and 2) prevention, reducing risk, delaying the onset of Alzheimer's or even preventing it altogether. The current diagnosis of Alzheimer's largely is based on symptoms and measuring mental decline. The issue with this approach is that by the time the disease is diagnosed, severe brain damage may already have occurred.

There is a lot of research being done into the early detection of Alzheimer's:

Identifying biomarkers: Biological markers or biomarkers, in short, are a definite way to determine the presence of a disease. For example, fasting blood glucose level for diabetes or blood tests for cholesterol. Some of the biomarkers being studied such as beta-amyloid and tau levels in cerebrospinal fluid.

Brain imaging: This is another research area for early detection. While there are some FDA approved imaging products in the market, there is a lot more research going on in the following three imaging technologies:

Structural imaging: Magnetic Resonance Imaging (MRI) and Computed Tomography (CT) can provide information about the shape, position, and volume of brain tissue and can possibly indicate brain shrinkage in specific areas of the brain that can shed light into the state of the disease.

Functional Imaging: In this type of imaging, functional wellness as well as the use of nutrients and other essential cell foods (sugar, oxygen) in various areas of the brain is assessed. These imaging techniques include positron emission tomography (PET) and functional MRI (fMRI).

Molecular Imaging: In this type of imaging, targeted radiotracers are used to detect brain cell and tissue changes. This technology includes PET, fMRI and single proton emission computed tomography (SPECT)

All these researches are making significant progress towards early detection and treatment.

CHAPTER 3. PREVENTION

In this chapter, we examine the various ways to reduce the risk of Alzheimer's (as well as other forms of dementia). Most of these prevention methods rely on lifestyle changes. By consciously taking an approach to keep your body and brain fit every day, one can prevent the symptoms, delay the onset, slow down progression, and completely prevent or even reverse the progress of the disease.

WHO SHOULD FOCUS ON PREVENTION?

Anyone who has witnessed a loved one go through the various stages of Alzheimer's knows how frightening the prospect of Alzheimer's is. As I stated earlier, anyone over the age of 65 is at risk, and the risk level doubles with every 5 years above 65. The earlier one starts making lifestyle changes, the better it is to delay the onset, reduce risk, or even prevent the disease. If you have someone in your family diagnosed with Alzheimer's, then the risk is even higher.

PREVENTION STEP #1: REGULAR EXERCISE & PHYSICAL ACTIVITY

Being physically active has many benefits, from reducing the risk of heart disease to preventing cancer, to preventing or reducing the risk of Alzheimer's. According to Alzheimer's Research and Prevention Foundation, regular physical activity can reduce the risk of developing Alzheimer's up to 50 percent. It is also shown that exercise can slow the progression of disease in those individuals who are already diagnosed with Alzheimer's.

One does not need to spend hours in the gym every day to get benefits but 30 minutes a day will do the job. It is important, though, to come up with an exercise plan and stick to it every day. The ideal plan includes both cardio exercise and strength training. Besides these, a good beginner plan will include walking or swimming for 30 minutes or more a day.

For those people with a lot of time on their hands, especially after retirement, picking up a physical activity such as senior league for sports or even gardening can help. The key is to do these activities regularly.

Besides these, strength/resistance and weight training help you maintain not only your muscles but brain health as well. Add 2-3 weight sessions of 20-30 minutes into your weekly routine.

Another physical activity is to take up yoga or tai chi. Both of these not only help with strengthening your body and improving flexibility but sharpen your mind and improve concentration as well. These exercises also help improve your balance, which is key as we age to prevent falls and risk of head injuries that can potentially increase the risk for Alzheimer's.

It is never too late to start an exercise regimen and even small things count. The key is to get you on your feet. Doing household chores such as vacuuming and doing dishes also counts. Even when you need to work at a desk or watch TV, standing up to work or watch TV will be more beneficial than sitting for a majority of the time.

PREVENTION STEP #2: MENTAL STIMULATION

Several studies have been conducted that concluded that people keeping mentally active through learning new things, solving problems, playing strategy games, etc. have had a lower risk of cognitive decline and Alzheimer's disease. This may be because mental stimulation through learning or strategy games strengthens the nerve cells and connections within the brain. In the NIH ACTIVE study (National Institute of Health ACTIVE study), older adults who received 10 sessions of mental training not only improved their cognitive score but continued to show long-lasting effects several years later.

The best mental stimulations involve not only problem solving but organization, planning, interaction, and communication.

Here are the recommendations on mental stimulation:

- Learn something new. Learn a new game, a language, a musical instrument, a science or technology topic. The greater the challenge, the greater the benefit. Be a lifelong learner.

- Strategy games, puzzles, and riddles.

    ○ Practice chess or other board games. Play with a partner instead of a computer whenever possible. The interaction helps.

- Play other games such as sudoku, scrabble, ken-ken, crossword puzzles, or cards.

- Play with other people whenever possible, such as at cards, scrabble, etc. Social interaction along with mental stimulation gives added benefit.

- Play brain teasers and trivia games.

- Make this a habit. Play some of these games with kids or grandkids every week.

- Keep a diary or journal to write down daily experiences of "who, what, where, when, and why". The process of writing things down helps to improve memory. Describe as vividly as possible. Visualize the events before writing them down.

- Practice memorization. Take it up as a hobby. Try to remember names, numbers (phone number, credit card number), and facts (state names, country names, capitals). Visualize and associate names with people and objects.

- Take up a new hobby. This could be learning and picking up a new game such as tennis, or something around the house such as gardening. This has the benefit of both mental and physical stimulation.

PREVENTION STEP #3: SOCIAL ENGAGEMENT

Humans are highly social animals. We thrive in a social or community setting. Our brains are wired for interacting with other people, animals, and nature. Staying socially engaged will reduce the risk of Alzheimer's in later stages of life, not to mention having people to care for you. Remaining socially active is even more important once you retire from active jobs.

Here are some recommendations:

- Volunteer in a church, temple, synagogue or mosque, or any other religious or non-profit entity.

- Join a club or social group of likeminded people (bingo club, cards club, or even a senior tennis club, that meets at least once a week). The key is to be active with the group regularly.

- Take up group lessons or a group learning activity (swim lessons, community college for a foreign language, musical instrument, gym lessons).

- Connect using a social network such as Facebook, Pinterest, Twitter, or Snapchat. One does not need to be on all social media platforms but having a platform to interact in the real or virtual world helps you keep engaged and connected.

- Make it a point to meet with friends at least once a week. This could be a coffee, lunch, or dinner date. Or it could be movies or a morning/weekend walk in the park. The key is to create a routine and stick with it.

- Make it a point to go out of the house. Find your special interests – in movies, museums, or libraries.

- Connect with your neighbors, get to know them.

- Find a social cause to be involved in.

- Plan and participate in family/social rituals, traditions, and celebrations.

- Write a book on your life experiences, you may have plenty of stories to tell the world.

PREVENTION STEP #4: HEART & HEAD CONNECTION

There is a very direct connection between heart health and brain health. Conditions that are known to decrease heart health, such as high blood pressure, diabetes, and high cholesterol, also increase the risk of Alzheimer's. Some studies have shown that 80 percent of Alzheimer's patients also have cardiovascular disease.

On the other hand, some of the autopsy studies have also shown that while some individuals had tau tangles and beta-amyloid plaques in their brains, they did not exhibit symptoms of Alzheimer's. Cardiovascular health may be the key factor in Alzheimer's and some researchers are working on the link between the two.

In short, anything heart-healthy (food, exercise) is also good for your brain and hence help prevent Alzheimer's.

As discussed in the prevention step #2, exercise helps to improve blood flow and has many cardiovascular benefits. The same benefits help with Alzheimer's, as exercise helps increase blood flow and oxygen in the brain and keeps the brain cells healthy.

PREVENTION STEP #5: STRESS MANAGEMENT

Stress is a cause for many ailments, most notably heart disease. Persistent stress also has a big toll on the brain and can cause brain shrinkage leading to Alzheimer's. While we know stress has an impact on heart conditions, we don't think much about stress impacting the brain. Keep in mind the strong heart to head connection. Anything bad for the heart is bad for the brain, too.

Below are some techniques for stress management:

Breathing

Breathing is one of the "in the moment" stress management techniques.

- Deep breathing. Take some deep breaths. With each deep breath, the body relaxes progressively.

- Abdominal breathing. Place hands on belly. Hands should go out with your belly on the inhale, in on the exhale. Repeat until feeling relaxed.

- Breath counting. 5 seconds of inhaling followed by 5 seconds of exhaling. Also, you can hold your breath for 5 seconds before exhaling.

Channel your inner peace

- Practice regular meditation.

- Practice daily prayer.

- Regular religious practice. Attending church service, going to temple, synagogue, or mosque.

Schedule daily relaxation techniques

- Practice yoga or tai chi.

Exercise helps reduce stress

- Pick up a game or a regular activity

- Try exercising or gym activities.

- Take up swimming.

- Try routinely running or walking.

Take time out for vacation

- All work and no play increases stress levels. Take time out. Schedule vacation time with friends or family.

Sense of humor/ laughing out loud

- Watch comedy films or shows.

- Try joking with friends and family.

- Or just laugh out loud for no reason.

Adopt a pet

- Pets help reduce stress.

- They also provide companionship.

PREVENTION STEP #6: A GOOD NIGHT'S SLEEP

As you have heard, sleep time is used by the brain for memory formation. The whole body uses sleep as a restorative process to recover from all the work the body did during waking hours. New research has shown that lack of sleep can increase the risk for many diseases including Alzheimer's. Some studies have shown the need for proper (REM stage) sleep for flushing out toxins from the brain. Poor sleep can cause the formation of beta-amyloid plaques in the brain that increases the risk for Alzheimer's.

Tips for sound sleep:

- Establish a regular schedule for sleep. A regular sleep cycle reinforces the body's natural clock and helps you to have a better sleep.

- Establish a routine and mood. A glass of warm milk, a hot bath, stretching, diary or journal entries, or dim lights may help.

- Switch off electronics – phones, laptops, TVs, etc. are huge distractions and impediments to sound sleep.

- Relax. If you are stressed it is hard to sleep. Use one of the relaxation techniques to decompress before sleep.

- Snoring or sleep apnea. Get tested and treated. It can make a huge difference in sleep quality.

PREVENTION STEP #7: PROTECT YOUR HEAD

Protect your head from head trauma. Head trauma that involves concussions is considered an Alzheimer's risk. You can reduce the risk by taking steps to protect your head in situations that can cause a head injury.

- Wear a seat belt in automobiles.

- Use a helmet as appropriate while participating in sports.

- Use a helmet when riding bikes.

- Make sure your home is "fall-proof". This is quite important as you get older. Falling in the shower or on steps are common causes of head injuries at home.

PREVENTION STEP#8: TAKE CARE OF YOUR TEETH AND GUMS

One may wonder how caring for your teeth has anything to do with Alzheimer's. Your teeth and brain are both housed in the head. Scientists have recently found that periodontal disease in which an inflammatory condition that could result in loss of teeth can indeed incite the start of Alzheimer's. A recent research conducted in the University of Chicago, Illinois found that mice that were infected with bacteria that cause gum disease had inflammation and deterioration in the brain as well.

Oral health is not only important for Alzheimer's but some cancers such as HPV and also cardiovascular diseases. So, keeping your gums and teeth healthy reduces the risk for Alzheimer's as it reduces inflammation of gums and teeth transmitting to brain cells.

PREVENTION STEP #9: DIET

Diet is the last step in prevention but in my opinion, one of the most important steps. As with many other diseases including cancer and heart disease, diet plays an important part in Alzheimer's. There are studies conducted that suggest the strong link between other physical disorders or diseases and the diseases of the brain. Inflammation in the brain and oxidative damage to brain cells impact brain health.

Several studies have been conducted on the relationship between diet and Alzheimer's and found that eating the Mediterranean diet has significantly reduced the risk of cognitive impairment and Alzheimer's disease. Similarly, a South Asian diet that includes a lot of spices and herbs seems to help reduce the risk as well.

Studies have also shown that the DASH diet (Dietary Approaches to Stop Hypertension) has benefits for Alzheimer's patients. The DASH diet promotes fruits and vegetables, low-fat dairy products, whole grains, fish, nuts, and seeds.

Here are some recommendations on dieting:

- Avoid foods that cause inflammation such as sugars and refined carbs (white rice, white/bleached flour, pasta).

- Include anti-inflammatory foods (including spices and herbs) into the diet.

- Eat a lot of fish. Omega-3 fats containing DHA help prevent Alzheimer's and dementia by countering plaque formation. Include oily fishes like salmon, tuna, sardines, mackerel, trout, etc. in your diet.

- Eat a lot of fruits and vegetables, especially colorful vegetables.

- Include the Mediterranean diet as part of your diet regiment.

- Practice the DASH diet.

- Eat whole foods and grains.

- Drink more tea.

- Eat more nuts and seeds.

- Avoid fast foods, fried foods, and packaged foods.

- Avoid processed foods.

- Eat foods that strengthen your digestive system and consequently improve your immunity.

- Eat fresh meals.

- Cook at home.

This author believes diet (along with exercise) is the most important prevention step. This conclusion is further strengthened by the worldwide Alzheimer's statistics. South Asian and Mediterranean countries have a much lower (India's is 100 times lower than the US) Alzheimer's incident rate compared to the western countries. South Asian countries hardly eat processed foods but eat more vegetables and use a lot more spices and herbs. These countries also have more social and family ties than some

of the developed countries. The next chapters are dedicated to Alzheimer's diet and recipes.

CHAPTER 4. BRAIN HEALTHY FOODS

As we age, the various cells in our bodies, including within the brain, age with us. We can observe the old age in people by looking at their face and body – sagging muscles, wrinkled skin, etc. The same is true for the brain; there are shrinkages and dead cells in the brain, too. Studies have shown that by incorporating superfoods and smart foods, one can increase the chances of arresting, maintaining, or even reversing the aging of both body and brain.

Below are four main characteristics of the foods that help maintain a healthy brain and provide neuroprotection.

ANTI-INFLAMMATORY PROPERTIES

Inflammation plays an important role in the natural healing process of the human body. It helps to defend against harmful invaders in our bodies such as bacteria that cause infection. Inflammation also helps the body carry out wound repair. Without inflammation, foreign invaders could cause damage to our bodies and ultimately kill us.

While short term, controlled inflammation is beneficial, it can become a major problem when it becomes chronic, such as arthritis. Chronic inflammation plays a major role in many serious health conditions such as heart disease, cancer, autoimmune diseases, Alzheimer's, and other various degenerative conditions.

Therefore, it is very important that inflammation is contained, and chronic inflammation is fought with medicines, supplements, foods, or through a combination of all in order to reduce or prevent it from happening. Most anti-inflammatory foods are, therefore, brain-healthy foods. By fighting inflammation that weakens the body's immune system and damages cells, these foods help improve the body's defenses against Alzheimer's and other diseases.

ANTIOXIDANT PROPERTIES

Oxidative damage caused by free radicals (highly reactive molecules with unpaired electrons) contributes to the risk of cancers, heart disease, diabetes, and Alzheimer's as well as age-related macular degeneration. Free radicals tend to react with important organic substances, such as fatty acids, proteins, or DNA, causing oxidative damage.

Antioxidants help neutralize free radicals and reduce the risk of oxidative damage. They "clean up" free radicals by interacting and forming harmless substances, thereby protecting healthy cells. There are several vitamins and supplements that are known to have antioxidant properties such as vitamins C and E and beta carotene. Many of the fruits (berries, grapes, etc.) and vegetables (kale, artichokes, bell pepper, etc.) contain antioxidants. Nuts such as walnuts and beverages such as tea and coffee also contain antioxidants. Antioxidants are often added to packaged food products to keep them from interacting with air.

By incorporating foods that have antioxidant properties, one can help reduce cell damage to the body and brain.

HEART HEALTH

As we have seen there is a strong connection between cardiovascular health and Alzheimer's disease. Foods that help reduce cholesterol and hypertension and improve circulation do indirectly help prevent Alzheimer's disease as well.

IMMUNE SYSTEM AND INFECTIONS

Foods that have the capability to fight infections, boost the immune system, and strengthen your gut are key in fighting many health conditions. A body that is weak in its defenses against foreign invaders is always at high risk for cancer, Alzheimer's, and many other diseases. Some of the recipes described in the next section use spices that are known to boost the immune system and help maintain a healthy digestive system. A significant part of the body's immunity results from a healthy gut, and thus maintaining a healthy digestive system enhances the body's overall immunity and helps reduce the risk of diseases.

The next several sections describe various foods that improve brain health and prevent Alzheimer's.

BRAIN FOOD #1: BERRIES

All berries are rich in antioxidants, which help neutralize free radicals in the body that usually cause cell damage. Cell damage in the brain due to oxidative stress is considered one of the reasons for Alzheimer's and dementia.

The main phytochemicals in berries are called anthocyanins. These antioxidants can counteract and neutralize free radicals. Berries are rich in other nutrients such as vitamin C, fiber, and minerals which can also fight brain cell damage.

The recommended list:

- Blueberries
- Blackberries
- Raspberries
- Strawberries
- Acai berries
- Goji berries
- Cherries

While all berries are rich in antioxidants, **blueberries** are especially good for the brain.

Suggestions:
Eat them raw. Add them to smoothies or juice them. Make sure to wash them thoroughly before cating.

BRAIN FOOD #2: NUTS & SEEDS

If you have not incorporated nuts and seeds into your diet, you should seriously consider adding them. At least 2-3 handfuls of nuts and seeds a week will provide you immense benefits.

Walnuts are especially good for brain health. Nuts have Vitamin E and also omega-3 fatty acids that help protect you from Alzheimer's by improving cognitive function and mental alertness. Some of these nuts also help prevent heart disease.

The recommended list:

- Walnuts
- Pecans
- Almonds
- Brazil nuts
- Peanuts
- Cashews
- Flax seeds
- Chia seeds
- Hemp seeds
- Sunflower seeds
- Pumpkin seeds

Suggestions:
Make it point to eat a handful of seeds/nuts every day. Walnuts are especially good for you. Replace your unhealthful snacks with nuts and seeds. Add them to smoothies. Top cereal bowls with nuts and berries. Snack on them instead of potato chips or other junk foods.

BRAIN FOOD #3: LEAFY GREENS

Dark leafy green vegetables have been getting more and more attention lately for their health benefits. Dark green leafy vegetables have a wide range of carotenoids such lutein and zeaxanthin, along with saponins and flavonoids in addition to vitamin A and K. A study conducted on the older population found that people who consumed at least one serving a day of leafy vegetables experienced slower mental decline than those who ate no vegetables.

The recommended list:

- Kale (all types – green, red, Lacinato)
- Spinach
- Chard
- Collard greens
- Mustard greens

Suggestions:
Make them part of smoothies and salads. Sauté them with onions, garlic, ginger, etc. Add some turmeric and coconut powder. Cream them or toss some chopped greens into your meat preparations. Kale is especially good and contains 600 percent of the daily allowance of vitamins A and K in one cup.

BRAIN FOOD #4: TEA

The antioxidant chemicals (catechins) in teas have the ability to scavenge for free radicals in the body and neutralize them. Tea, with its antioxidant properties and a modest amount of caffeine, can help maintain focus and enhance memory and mood. Of all the tea varieties, **green tea** offers the most promise and according to some researchers, catechins can block amyloid plaque formation.

The recommended list:

- Green tea
- Black tea

- Chamomile tea
- Dandelion tea
- Essiac tea

Suggestions:
Make a couple of cups of tea a day as part of your daily routine. Drink freshly brewed instead of store bought (which probably is not beneficial and often contains too much sugar).

BRAIN FOOD #5: COFFEE

Coffee improves focus and helps boost memory. A Harvard study found that people who drink 3-5 cups of coffee daily have a lower risk of developing neurological diseases. Coffee contains an anti-inflammatory substance called chlorogenic acid which helps counter chronic inflammation.

BRAIN FOOD #6: HEALTHFUL UNREFINED OILS – OLIVE OIL & COCONUT OIL

Using unrefined oils such as coconut oil and extra virgin olive oil instead of refined oils can help improve the immune system. Cod liver oil (taken by the spoonful as a supplement) also has great health benefits. They all also have Omega-3 fatty acids that can help nourish the cells in your body and keep them healthy, prevent oxidation, and improve your brain function.

Coconut oil could be especially beneficial against Alzheimer's as coconut oil contains MCT or medium-chain triglycerides. MCTs are shorter fatty acid chains compared to long-chain triglycerides (LCT). MCTs are absorbed by the liver and transform them into ketones. As some researches have shown, ketones may have beneficial effects on brain function to help reduce Alzheimer's symptoms.

Suggestions:
Use these unrefined oils for cooking, baking, and making salad dressings.

BRAIN FOOD #7: DARK CHOCOLATE

Dark chocolate has powerful antioxidant and anti-inflammatory properties. It contains several natural brain-boosting compounds including small amounts of caffeine. Caffeine improves focus, concentration, and mood by stimulating the production of endorphins.

Suggestions:
Remember that only unprocessed or minimally processed dark chocolate (at least 70% cocoa) provides these benefits. Milk chocolates and white chocolates that you buy from the supermarket are usually heavily processed and do not provide the same benefits. An ounce of dark chocolate a day can provide immense benefits to improving brain health.

BRAIN FOOD #8: AVOCADOS

Avocados contain many essential nutrients such as vitamin B, vitamin C, vitamin K, and **folate.** In addition, avocados contain "good" fat that helps to stabilize blood sugar levels. Overall, these nutrients in avocados improve cognitive function, memory, and focus. Avocados also help prevent blood clots and protect against stroke.

Suggestions:
Include avocados in your daily salads, guacamole, or as part of breakfast.

BRAIN FOOD #9: BROCCOLI

Broccoli contains high vitamin K and **choline** that will help improve memory and focus. It also contains high levels of vitamin C and fiber. It is a superfood that is great for preventing both cancer and Alzheimer's

BRAIN FOOD #10: EGGS

Eggs contain several nutrients that are important for brain health such as vitamins B6, B12, **folate,** and **choline.** All of these are very important nutrients for brain health and eggs are the easiest way to get them in your diet.

BRAIN FOOD #11: COLORFUL FRUITS & VEGGIES

One of the oft-made suggestions for healthy eating is the notion of "eating the colors of the rainbow." Brightly colored vegetables and fruits carry abundant phytochemicals that are full of carotenoid antioxidants and other essential vitamins.

Beta-carotene is one of the many carotenoids found in colored vegetables. It has been studied and found to have benefits in fighting cancers of the eye, skin, and other vital organs in the body besides being helpful in detoxification and the boosting of the immune system.

Below are some common fruits and vegetables that are colorful which should find a way into one's daily diet plans. Many of these foods have been shown to fight several cancers such as stomach, ovarian, breast, and lung cancers.

Pink/Red – Tomatoes, watermelon, red chard, pomegranate, cherries, strawberries, apples, bell peppers, raspberries, and grapefruit.

Blue/Purple – Eggplant, grapes, beets, red cabbage, purple cauliflower, blueberries, and prunes.

Yellow/Orange – Orange, apricots, papaya, mango, banana, pineapple, carrot, pumpkins, and squash.

Green – Bright green leafy vegetables - kale, spinach, peppers, celery, and artichokes.

Suggestions:
Make it a point to eat one or two servings of colored vegetables/fruits a day. Fruits may be part of smoothies; vegetables may be combined with other spices/herbs or eaten as part of a salad.

Brain Food #12: Oily Fish

The body needs essential fatty acids such as omega-3 fatty acids EPA (eicosapentaenoic acid) and DHA (docosahexaenoic acid), and oily deep-water fish are the best naturally occurring and easy to absorb source of these fatty acids. These are very important for the body's general wellbeing but especially so for the brain, heart, and joints. Some studies have linked low DHA levels to increased risk of dementia, memory loss, and Alzheimer's.

Oily fishes such as salmon, trout, mackerel, sardines, and herring are excellent sources of omega-3 essential acids. According to a study conducted by Tufts University in Boston, participants who ate at least 3 servings of oily fish a week had a 50% lower risk of Alzheimer's disease and dementia.

The fish, caught wild, have more omega-3 and fewer toxins than farmed fish. So, buy wild-caught versions of these fish whenever possible.

While some nuts and seeds (also good brain foods) such as walnuts, flaxseeds, etc. also are rich in omega-3, they lack the EPA and DHA components in a readily available form for the body to absorb compared to the oily fishes.

Suggestions:

Consume 2-3 servings of wild-caught salmon, sardines or other oily fish every week.

BRAIN FOOD #13: FERMENTED FOODS

Fermented foods do not directly boost memory, concentration or brain health. But a healthier gut or digestive system is greatly important for overall health, improved immunity, and increased ability to fight inflammation and diseases including

Alzheimer's. This is the reason for including the group of fermented foods in this section.

There are trillions of microorganisms living in our bodies. Most of them live in our gut or digestive system. These "good bacteria" living in our gut contribute to digestion, helps improve immunity, and are hugely important to maintaining our health and our bodies' ability to fight disease.

Fermented foods are rich in probiotics and eating fermented food is a sure way to improve immunity and help digestion.

The recommended list:

- Yogurt – provides billions of probiotic cultures
- Kefir – fermented milk drink abundant in probiotics
- Kombucha - fermented tea
- Raw non-pasteurized cheese – provides active cultures
- Sauerkraut – made of fermented cabbage
- Kimchi – Korean version of sauerkraut; fermented vegetables including cabbage
- Pickles – pickle anything and it is good for your gut
- Miso – made of fermented soybeans with barley/brown rice and koji; a traditional Japanese dish/seasoning
- Tempeh – a fermented soybeans product; a traditional soybean product of Indonesia

Suggestions:
Include 2-3 servings of one or more of the fermented foods in your diet a week.

BRAIN FOOD #14: SPICES

There are many spices that have significant anti-inflammatory and antioxidant capabilities that are proven to be also neuroprotective. In this author's opinion, the top spices for neuroprotection are:

- Turmeric
- Cinnamon
- Ginger
- Garlic

Of course, there are other spices with anti-inflammatory and antioxidant properties that are good for the brain. But I consider these spices to be everyday spices that are easy to incorporate in everyday diets.

Turmeric

Turmeric is a well-known spice in Asian cooking, especially in South Asia. Turmeric comes from the root of the turmeric plant, which is part of the ginger family. The turmeric root is cleaned, dried, and ground to create the yellow turmeric powder. Turmeric is used as an herbal supplement, added to flavor food as part of curry powder or as a standalone spice, added to cosmetics, or used as a food coloring. Turmeric is also used as a skin treatment and beauty enhancer. Evidently, it has been used by humans for thousands of years and is a time-tested wonder.

Turmeric powder is bright yellow and provides a distinct yellow color to the Indian "curry powder." Turmeric has been one of the key ingredients in Asian cuisine for years.

The main active ingredient in turmeric is called curcumin, which has very powerful medicinal properties. However, there are two challenges in fully realizing the benefits of turmeric. First, the curcumin content is only about 3% of turmeric by weight. Second, curcumin is not easily absorbed by the body. Curcumin absorption can be substantially enhanced by consuming black pepper, which contains *piperine*, along with turmeric. Also, fatty foods have proven to aid curcumin absorption as well. To consume a sufficient dosage of curcumin, a combination of curcumin/turmeric extract supplements along with a diet prepared with turmeric is recommended.

Turmeric is a rich source of many essential vitamins and minerals; it does not contain any cholesterol but is an excellent source of antioxidants and dietary fiber, which helps to control bad cholesterol levels.

Fresh turmeric root is a very good source of vitamins such as vitamin C, vitamin B 6, vitamin E, and niacin. Turmeric is also a great source of several minerals such as calcium, iron, potassium, manganese, copper, zinc, and magnesium.

Turmeric's antioxidant levels are one of the highest among popular spices and herbs and are an excellent brain-boosting substance on many levels.

Ginger

Ginger (*Zingiber officinale*) is a flowering plant whose root is widely used as a spice and traditional medicine over thousands of years in Asia. Ginger belongs to the same family as turmeric and cardamom.

Ginger is widely used in Asian cooking, especially in China and India. While turmeric, which belongs to the same family as ginger, is mostly used in the powder form, ginger is used as a fresh ingredient in most cooking.

Ginger has been one of the key ingredients in Asian cuisine for centuries, especially used as part of meat recipes. When dried and ground, ginger results in a tan powder that is used in baking (gingerbread, cookies, crackers, cakes, etc.) and making beverages (ginger ale, ginger beer, etc.). Ginger, either powdered or fresh, can be used in teas and is an essential component of 'masala chai'.

The main bioactive active ingredient in ginger is called gingerol and it has very powerful medicinal properties, including antioxidant and anti-inflammatory properties. Ginger is used in several alternative/traditional medicines in the East.

Garlic

Garlic is part of the *Allium* (onion) family and is closely related to shallots, onions, Chinese onions, chives, and leeks. There are 400+ varieties of garlic in the world today.

But beyond its sharp odor, garlic offers a number of health benefits. While most of the garlic production and consumption is in Asia, garlic is finding more and more uses in the west as part of cooking and health supplements.

The main active ingredient in garlic is called polysulphide allicin and is responsible primarily for its medicinal properties. This compound, allicin, formed when garlic cloves are chopped or crushed, not only provides the medicinal properties but the distinct taste and smell as well.

Garlic is extremely nutritious and is a source of vitamins C and B6, along with the minerals manganese and selenium. Garlic also contains minor amounts of other minerals such as calcium, copper, potassium, phosphorous, and iron.

Just three cloves of garlic (about 9 grams) a day provide a recommended daily value of 8% manganese, 7% vitamin B6, 4% vitamin C, 3% copper, 3% selenium, and 2% each phosphorous, calcium and vitamin B1. Many of these nutrients are good for your overall health.

Cinnamon

Cinnamon is not only nutrient-rich but also has many health benefits. Ancient humans were attracted to cinnamon due to its sweetness and perfume and soon realized the many health benefits. Cinnamon was used in Ayurveda as a remedy for toothache, respiratory tract infections, chest congestion, stomach ailments, and cold and flu. Cinnamon's antibacterial, anti-viral, and antifungal properties were used in food preservation to make sure the harvest is not spoiled.

Many of the recent studies, while confirming the benefits ancient civilizations identified, have found several additional health benefits such as antioxidant, anti-inflammatory, and anticoagulant properties, as well as reducing cholesterol and blood sugar levels. Other studies have found benefits such as slowing down cognitive decline, HIV treatment, and anti-cancer properties.

Cinnamon is known to have one of the highest antioxidant rates among the many commonly used foods. In a study of 26 common spices and herbs on their antioxidant properties, cinnamon came out on top eclipsing garlic, oregano, thyme, and cloves.

Compounds in cinnamon are being studied for their ability to stop the buildup of tau proteins that cause tangles in the brain, which are considered a precursor to Alzheimer's.

BRAIN FOOD #15: HERBS

Like spices, a number of herbs also have neuroprotective properties. The most significant among them are:

- Rosemary
- Sage
- Ginkgo Biloba
- Lion's Mane
- Bacopa Monnieri or Brahmi
- Ashwagandha
- Ginseng

- Gotu Kola or Indian Pennywort
- Lemon balm

Rosemary has neurogenerative properties like many other herbs. The main ingredient in rosemary, called carnosic acid, neutralizes free radicals in the brain and helps improve brain health, fight against strokes, fight Alzheimer's and arrest the aging of the brain.

Sage is considered to possess memory-enhancing properties and likely to be beneficial for Alzheimer's patients based on evidence-based studies. Rosemary and sage may be added to roasted chicken, tomato sauce and soups.

Ginkgo biloba is commonly used as a treatment for dementia in Chinese traditional medicine. Gingko biloba may improve cognitive function by stimulating blood flow to the brain.

Lion's Mane is a white shaggy mushroom that resembles a lion's mane. Lion's Mane is used in ancient Chinese medicine and may improve cognitive function, prevent memory loss, and reduce symptoms of depression and anxiety, among other benefits.

Bacopa Monnieri or Brahmi is used in traditional Ayurvedic medicine for its cognition and memory enhancing properties. A 2001 study found that Brahmi significantly improved learning and memory retention over placebo.

Ashwagandha is an ayurvedic herb that may help the aging brain in a couple of ways – 1) inhibit the formation of beta-amyloid plaques and 2) prevent oxidative damage to brain cells.

Ginseng, one of the most popular herbs in Chinese medicine, contains anti-inflammatory compounds called ginsenosides which have shown to reduce the beta-amyloid build up in the brain.

The best way to consume ginkgo biloba, lion's mane, ashwagandha, and ginseng are through extracts and supplements. Extracts, supplements, and tea formulations of these ancient herbs are available in many online stores including Amazon.

Gotu Kola is used in both Chinese traditional medicine and Ayurveda to improve mental clarity. Some animal studies have shown that this herb may also help fight oxidative damage to brain cells.

Lemon balm is often taking in tea form can help reduce anxiety and improve sleep function. Lemon balm may help improve cognition.

BRAIN FOOD #16: BONE BROTH

Bone broth is considered a new age miracle drink. It is gaining popularity with athletes and celebrities as a wellness drink. By combining the immense benefits of nutrients and minerals in traditional bone broth with the medicinal properties of spices and herbs, we can make an even more potent and healthful drink. Below are some of the benefits of these spicy bone broths:

Antioxidant: Contents in bone broth such as glycine and gelatin both contain antioxidants which, coupled with antioxidants in spices such as turmeric and ginger, make bone broth one of the best sources of antioxidants. As noted in my other books, antioxidants fight free radicals (which cause cancer and other debilitating diseases).

Anti-inflammatory: By adding ginger, garlic, and turmeric in the preparation of bone broth, one enhances the anti-inflammatory properties of the broth.

Detoxification: Bone broth made by adding vegetables that contain sulfur helps the body to manufacture detox agents such as glutathione (amino acid). These detox agents help your kidneys to detox heavy metals from the body.

Bone health: Bone broth is an excellent source of calcium, magnesium, and phosphorous, which help bones to stay strong and healthy.

Fight infections: As a result of enhanced immunity and a strong digestive system, bone broth helps fight infections.

Improves immunity: Minerals and amino acids in bone broth help improve the immune system.

Speedy recovery: With so many benefits such as boosting the immune system, improving the digestive system, and fighting infection, it is no wonder bone broth helps in speedy recovery of the body from common ailments.

Gut cleaning: Bone broth helps proper digestion of food and keeps your gut and digestive system healthy.

Improves joints: Bone broth contains glucosamine and chondroitin, which help to maintain joints and keep them healthy and strong.

Helps athletic performance: Healthy joints and bones help improve your athleticism and reduce joint pain after exercise.

Improves metabolism and helps weight loss: An improved digestive system and a healthy gut help promote proper metabolism and weight loss.

Beauty enhancer: Collagen in bone broth helps skin, hair, and nails to be healthy and shiny.

As you see from the above benefits, when combined with healthful vegetables and medicinal spices and herbs, bone broth indeed becomes a miracle drink that improves your health, boosts immunity, fights diseases, and keeps you feeling young.

5. BRAIN NOURISHING RECIPE IDEAS

As we discussed in the introductory chapter, Finland and the US have the highest Alzheimer's rates at 54 and 46 respectively per 100,000 people. For the same size population, India has 0.46 (100 times less than the US) and the Mediterranean region has about 1.5 (30 times less than the US). This is no coincidence but attributable to several lifestyles and diet differences between them:

- Freshly cooked meals instead of processed foods

- No or little fast foods

- More vegetables than meat in the diet

- Use of healthful spices and herbs in cooking

- Stronger social and family bonds

As one can see, healthy eating and diet choices are probably the most important factors attributable to lower Alzheimer's incident rates. This chapter focuses on fresh and healthy cooking using some of the best Alzheimer's fighting ingredients identified in previous chapters.

TEAS

As described earlier, teas help prevent Alzheimer's. The recipes below combine transitional tea with brain boosting and Alzheimer's fighting spices such as turmeric, ginger, cinnamon, and garlic.

Turmeric, ginger, and garlic may be used to make drinks such as teas, smoothies, and other drinks. There are several ways to make teas with ginger and turmeric. Fresh turmeric or ginger root may be added to smoothies along with other fruits or vegetables. While making smoothies, remember that adding a pinch of black pepper or fat such as coconut oil or flaxseed oil helps the absorption of curcumin, turmeric's active ingredient.

BASIC TURMERIC TEA

Ingredients:

- ½ - 2 teaspoon turmeric powder or ½ inch – 2 inches long fresh turmeric root, grated (start with ½ teaspoon and increase the amount as you develop a taste for turmeric)
- 1 tsp honey (or to taste)
- Pinch freshly ground black pepper or pepper powder
- 1-2 cups water

Method

1. Put the turmeric and ground pepper in a cup or pot, add one spoon of water, mix and make it into a paste.

2. Boil 1-2 cups of water and add to the turmeric paste. Mix it well.
3. Strain out the turmeric pieces, if any.
4. Let it cool for a couple of minutes and add honey. Enjoy warm.

BASIC GINGER TEA

Ingredients:

- ½-2 inches fresh ginger, grated
- 1 tsp honey (or to taste)
- 1 tsp fresh lemon juice
- 1-2 cups water

Method

1. Add grated ginger to water and boil it for a couple of minutes.
2. Let it cool for a couple of minutes.
3. Filter ginger out; add honey and lemon juice; stir and enjoy lukewarm.

BLACK TEA WITH GINGER AND CARDAMOM

Basic Ingredients:

- ½-1-inch fresh ginger peeled and sliced/crushed
- 1 tsp honey (or to taste)
- 1-2 cups water
- 1 black tea bag

Optional Ingredients

- ½ teaspoon lemon juice
- 2 cardamom pods

Method

1. Add the ginger slices and optional cardamom to 1-2 cups of water and boil.
2. Add the black tea bag.
3. Let it cool for a couple of minutes.
4. Remove tea bag, filter ginger slices; add honey and optional lemon, and enjoy warm.

TURMERIC TEA WITH GINGER

Ingredients

- ½ - 2 teaspoons turmeric powder or ½ inch – 2 inches long fresh turmeric root, grated
- ½ inch – 1 inch fresh ginger, grated or thinly sliced
- 1 tsp honey (or to taste)
- Pinch freshly ground black pepper or pepper powder
- 1-2 cups water

Method

1. Put the turmeric, ground pepper, and ginger in a cup or pot and add one spoon of water, mix and make it a paste.
2. Boil 1-2 cups of water and add to the turmeric and ginger paste. Mix it well.

3. Strain out the ginger/turmeric pieces. Let it cool for a couple of minutes, add honey, and enjoy warm.

GREEN TEA WITH TURMERIC AND GINGER

Ingredients

- ½ - 2 teaspoons turmeric powder or ½ inch – 2 inches long fresh turmeric root
- ½ inch – 1 inch fresh ginger, grated or thinly sliced
- 1 tsp honey (or to taste)
- 1 pinch freshly ground black pepper or pepper powder
- 1-2 cups of green tea

Method

1. Process turmeric, ginger, and black pepper in a blender until smooth.
2. Add the hot green tea, mix well.
3. Filter if needed. Add honey and enjoy

Note:

If using fresh turmeric root, either grind it as part of the rest of the ingredients or boil the root in 1-2 cups of water and green tea for 5 minutes on low heat. Then add pepper and honey once it cools down.

MASALA CHAI (SPICED TEA)

There are several ways to make masala chai. When I make it, I only use ginger and cardamom. The other ingredients to add based on one's taste are cinnamon, cloves, pepper, and fennel seeds.

Basic Ingredients

- ½ inch – 1 inch fresh peeled ginger, grated or crushed
- 4-6 cardamoms, crushed
- 1 inch long cinnamon stick or ¼ tsp cinnamon powder
- ½ cup 2% milk
- 3 cups of water
- 2-4 tsp black tea or 2-3 tea bags

Optional Ingredients

- 2-4 cloves
- ¼ tsp pepper powder or about 4 peppercorns
- ¼ teaspoon fennel seeds
- 2-4 tsp brown sugar

Method

1. Grind or crush cardamom, cinnamon, cloves, fennel seeds, and pepper in a spice grinder or mortar.
2. In a pan, add the ground mix and ginger and pour in 3 cups of water. Mix it well and bring it to a boil.
3. Reduce heat and let it simmer for a minute or two.
4. Now add the tea, mix, and let it boil for one minute on low heat.
5. Add milk and sugar and mix well. Strain out all the ingredients and enjoy.

If you have not tried masala chai before, I suggest you start with ginger and cardamom and then introduce other items before settling on the ingredients you like best.

GINGER AND LEMON TEA

Ingredients

- ½ inch – 1 inch fresh ginger, grated or crushed
- ½ tsp lemon juice
- 1 tsp honey
- 2 cups of water

Method

1. Boil 2 cups of water in a saucepan.
2. Add ginger and let it boil for 2-3 minutes.
3. Remove from heat and add lemon. Add honey and enjoy warm

GARLIC TEA WITH GINGER AND LEMON

Basic Ingredients

- 1-2 cloves garlic, crushed
- ½ inch fresh ginger, grated or thinly sliced
- 1 tsp honey (or to taste)
- 1 tsp lemon juice
- 2 cups of water

Optional Ingredients

- Pinch black pepper powder
- 2 tsp apple cider vinegar

Method

1. Boil 2 cups of water and add crushed garlic and ginger; let it boil for 1 minute.
2. Add optional pepper and apple cider vinegar.
3. Switch off the heat and let it sit for 20 minutes.
4. Strain out the ginger/garlic pieces. Let it cool for a couple of minutes.
5. Add honey and lemon juice, and enjoy warm.

This drink is good for digestion, fighting cold/flu, clearing nasal congestion, sore throat, etc.

SMOOTHIES

TROPICAL SMOOTHIE

Basic Ingredients

- ½ - 2 teaspoons turmeric powder or ½ inch – 2 inches long fresh cleaned and sliced turmeric root (start with ½ tsp and increase the amount as you develop a taste for turmeric)
- ½ inch – 1 inch fresh ginger, grated or thinly sliced
- 1 pinch freshly ground black pepper or pepper powder
- 1 banana
- 1 cup pineapple, mango or papaya
- 1 cup milk or ½ cup plain yogurt
  ½ cup ice

Optional Ingredients

- 1 tsp honey (or to taste)

Method

Process all the ingredients in a blender until smooth.

GREEN SMOOTHIE WITH GARLIC, GINGER, AND TURMERIC

Basic Ingredients

- ½ - 2 teaspoons turmeric powder or ½ inch – 2 inches long fresh cleaned and sliced turmeric root
- ½ inch – 1 inch fresh ginger, grated or thinly sliced
- 1-2 cloves garlic
- 1 pinch freshly ground black pepper or pepper powder
- 1 cup kale, chopped
- 1 cup spinach
- 1-2 kiwis, peeled
- ½ cup blueberries
- 1-2 cups filtered water (coconut water may be used instead)
- ½ cup ice

Optional Ingredients

- ½ cup sliced cucumber
- ¼ avocado
- 1 tsp honey (or to taste)
- 3-4 mint leaves

Method

Process all the ingredients in a blender until smooth. Blueberries may be substituted with blackberries depending on your liking. Serves 3-4. By mixing and matching the "green" ingredients, you may try a couple of different green smoothies.

GOLDEN YELLOW SMOOTHIE

Ingredients

- ½ - 2 teaspoons turmeric powder or ½ inch – 2 inches long fresh cleaned and sliced turmeric root
- ½ inch – 1 inch fresh ginger, grated or thinly sliced
- 1 tsp coconut oil or butter
- 1 carrot, washed and cut into pieces
- 1 mango, peeled and sliced
- 1 cup orange or mango juice
- ½ cup ice

Optional Ingredients

- 1 tsp honey (or to taste)

Method

Process all the ingredients in a blender until smooth.

VERY BERRY SMOOTHIE

Ingredients

- ½ inch – 1 inch fresh ginger, grated or thinly sliced
- ½ cup blueberries
- ½ cup blackberries
- ½ cup raspberries
- ½ cup strawberries
- 1 cup 2% milk or low-fat yogurt
- ½ cup ice

Optional Ingredients

- 1 tsp honey (or to taste)

Method

Process all the ingredients in a blender until smooth.

GARLIC AND LEMON DRINK

Ingredients

- 3 full garlic bulbs (about 100gm), cloves peeled and chopped
- 4 organic lemons, washed and chopped
- 3-4 cups water

Optional Ingredients

- 4-5 tsp honey

Method

1. Add garlic and lemons to boiling water and keep it boiling on low heat for 15 minutes.
2. Switch off the heat and let it cool down. Add honey and refrigerate in a glass jar.

Drink 3 tablespoons daily until the drink is finished. Take a 2-3 week pause before making and consuming this again.

Note:

This is an adapted recipe from www.healthyfoodteam.com. This is a natural remedy against cancer-causing bad cells, helping to improve cholesterol and clearing clogged arteries.

Broths

VEGAN BROTH

This is a simple broth that provides healing and helps with minor ailments such as cold and flu. This is fully vegan and contains nutrients from a number of vegetables and herbs.

Ingredients

- 2-3 celery sticks, cut into inch pieces
- 3 medium tomatoes, chopped
- 1 bell pepper, cut into pieces
- 1 large onion, peeled and cut into pieces
- 1 pound (2-3 medium) carrots, washed cut into pieces
- 1 cup kale
- 1 medium beetroot, washed and cut into pieces
- ½ cup parsley, chopped
- ½ cup cilantro, chopped
- 3-4 garlic cloves, crushed
- 3-4 whole cloves
- 5-6 black peppercorns or ½ tsp pepper powder
- 1-2 bay leaves
- 1 gallon water
- Salt to taste (if you must or avoid salt)

Method

1. Add everything to a large pot. Bring to a boil

2. Lower the heat, and simmer covered for about 1 hour. Stir occasionally.

3. Once the vegetables are cooked, strain the broth into a large bowl.

4. Add salt to taste, add some chopped fresh herbs of your choice, and serve warm.

5. Refrigerate any remaining broth.

6. The strained vegetables are pretty good and can be eaten separately or pureed in a blender as is.

SPICY VEGAN BROTH

This is a spicy version of the vegan broth that immediately precedes it. It helps with congestion, cold, flu, sore throat, and other ailments due to infections. Like the non-spicy version, this broth also is healing and easy on your gut. The antioxidants and anti-inflammatory compounds in turmeric and ginger make this broth even more healthful.

Ingredients – veggies

- 2-3 celery sticks, cut into inch pieces
- 3 medium tomatoes, chopped
- 1 bell green pepper, cut into pieces
- 1 red bell pepper, cut into pieces
- ¼ of a medium red cabbage, chopped
- 1 large onion, peeled and cut into 1 inch cubes
- ½ cup chopped onion (for sautéing)
- 1 pound (2-3 medium) carrots, washed and cut into pieces
- 1 cup kale
- 1 medium beetroot, washed and cut into pieces

Ingredients – spices and herbs

- ½ cup parsley, chopped

- ½ cup cilantro, chopped
- 3-4 garlic cloves, crushed
- 3-4 whole cloves
- 5-6 black peppercorns or ½ tsp pepper powder
- 1-2 bay leaves
- 1 inch ginger, finely chopped
- 2 tsp turmeric powder or 2 inches of fresh root
- 2 jalapeño peppers, sliced lengthwise (seed in or out depending on your heat tolerance)
- ½ tsp cayenne powder
- ½ tsp cumin powder

Ingredients – other

- 1 gallon water
- Salt to taste (if you must or avoid salt)
- 1 tsp coconut or vegetable oil

Method

1. In a medium pan, heat oil and add onion for sautéing, crushed garlic, ginger, and jalapeño peppers.

2. Sauté for 2-3 minutes or until the onion becomes translucent. Add all the remaining spices (cayenne, cumin, turmeric, cloves, bay leaves, pepper powder, etc.) and sauté for another 2-3 minutes so the spices are blended well (make sure not to burn them).

3. Transfer the spice mix into a large pot (add some water to wash out any remaining spice mix from the pan and pour it into the large pot.)

4. Add all the vegetables into the pot and add water; bring to a boil.

5. Lower the heat; simmer covered for about 1 hour. Stir occasionally.

6. Once the vegetables are cooked, strain the broth into a large bowl.

7. Add salt to taste, add some chopped fresh herbs of your choice, and serve warm.

8. Refrigerate any remaining broth.

The strained-out vegetables are also nutritious and may be consumed separately.

BONE BROTHS

Bone broth is considered a new age miracle drink. It is gaining popularity with athletes and celebrities as a wellness drink. By combining the immense benefits of nutrients and minerals in traditional bone broth with the medicinal properties of spices and herbs, we can make an even more potent and healthful drink. As explained in Chapter 4 on brain foods (Brain Food #16), there are numerous benefits for bone broth including anti-aging and brain health. When combined with healthful vegetables and medicinal spices and herbs, bone broth indeed becomes a miracle drink that improves your health, boosts immunity, fights diseases, and keeps you feeling young.

Bone Broth Recipes

As one can imagine, the main ingredient in bone broth is some type of bone; one can mix and match additional ingredients depending on your taste, the kind of flavor you like, and the level of spiciness you can tolerate. Usually, one or more of the following bones are used as part of the bone broth:

- Chicken

- Turkey

- Fish

- Beef

- Lamb or goat

- Pork

One has a large choice of vegetables.

- Carrots

- Celery

- Tomatoes

- Bell peppers – all colors

- Beets

- Onions

- Kale

- Red cabbage

- Lentils and beans

Spices and herbs

- Turmeric (powder or root)

- Ginger root

- Garlic

- Bay leaves

- Whole cloves

- Black peppercorns

- Curry powder

- Parsley

- Cilantro

- Thyme

- Rosemary

- Oregano

- Cumin seeds or cumin powder

- Fennel seeds or fennel powder

- Cinnamon

Others:

- Apple cider vinegar
- Filtered water

EASY BONE BROTH (CHICKEN)

This is one of the easiest ways to make bone broth. I make it out of the carcass from the rotisserie chicken bought from the departmental store. I remove all the meat and use it as a regular meal for the family and use the entire carcass (without the skins – but skins may be used as well if you prefer) for the bone broth. Not only is this method much simpler but also takes less time, as the chicken bones are already cooked.

Ingredients

- Chicken carcass from a full rotisserie chicken – skin and fat optional
- 4 celery sticks, cut into 1 inch pieces
- 3 medium tomatoes, chopped
- 1 bell pepper, cut into pieces (any color)
- 1 large onion, peeled and quartered
- 1 pound (2-3 medium) carrots, washed and cut into pieces
- ½ cup parsley, chopped
- ½ cup cilantro, chopped
- 3-4 garlic cloves, crushed
- 3-4 whole cloves
- 2 inches ginger, peeled and grated
- 5-6 black peppercorns or ½ tsp pepper powder
- 1-2 bay leaves
- 1 gallon water
- Salt to taste (if you must or avoid salt)

Optional Ingredients

- 2-3 Jalapeño peppers split lengthwise

Method

1. Add everything to a large pot. Bring to a boil
2. Lower the heat; simmer covered for about 2-3 hours.
3. Once the vegetables are fully cooked, strain the broth into a large bowl using a mesh strainer.

4. Add salt to taste, add some chopped fresh herbs of your choice, and serve warm.

5. Refrigerate any remaining broth.

Recipe Notes:

1. The strained vegetables are pretty good and can be eaten after removing all the bone pieces.

2. A slow cooker or pressure cooker may be used for cooking. A pressure cooker will reduce the cooking time if you are in a hurry.

3. You can make this broth a meal by making it a soup. For making it a soup – add ½ cup split lentils and ½ cup brown or white rice to the pot. Add some of the vegetables back and enjoy it when you are recovering from illness and you don't feel like having a full meal. It is very filling and nutritious. This is also a good meal when you are working on a weight loss program.

BONE BROTH (CHICKEN-SPICY)

This is a spicy version of the previous chicken bone broth. This spicy broth immediately helps with congestion, cold, flu, sore throat and other ailments due to infections. This broth also is healing and easy on your gut, besides all the long-term health benefits that come with regular consumption of this bone broth and these healing spices.

Basic Ingredients:

- 4 lb. chicken bones – any combination of wings, necks, and feet

- 4 celery sticks, cut into 1 inch pieces
- 3 medium tomatoes, chopped
- 1 bell pepper, cut into pieces (any color)
- 1 large onion, peeled and quartered
- 1 pound (2-3 medium) carrots, washed and cut into pieces
- 1 gallon water
- 2 tbsp raw unfiltered apple cider vinegar
- Salt to taste (if you must or avoid salt)

Ingredients – spices and herbs

- 2 tsp turmeric powder
- 1 tsp cumin powder or cumin seeds
- 1 tsp coriander powder
- 1 tsp cayenne powder
- 2 tsp fenugreek seeds
- ½ cup parsley, chopped
- ½ cup cilantro, chopped
- ½ cup rosemary
- 3-4 garlic cloves, crushed
- 3-4 whole cloves
- 2 inches ginger root, peeled and grated
- 5-6 black peppercorns or ½ tsp pepper powder
- 1-2 bay leaves

Optional Ingredients

- 2-3 Jalapeño peppers split lengthwise

Method

1. In a medium a pan, heat oil and crackle cumin seeds and fenugreek seeds. Add onion, crushed garlic, ginger, and jalapeño peppers.

2. Sauté for 2-3 minutes or until the onion becomes translucent. Add all the remaining spices (cayenne, cumin, turmeric, coriander, cloves, bay leaves, fenugreek, parsley, cilantro, rosemary, and pepper powder) and sauté for another 2-3 minutes so the spices are blended well and sufficiently roasted (make sure not to burn the spices).
3. Transfer the spice mix into a large pot (add some water to wash out any remaining spice mix from the pan and pour it into the large pot).
4. Add all chicken bones and vegetables into a large crock-pot and add water and apple cider vinegar and bring to a boil.
5. Lower the heat and simmer covered for 24-48 hours.
6. Once the bones and vegetables are cooked, strain the broth into a large bowl.
7. Add salt to taste, add some chopped fresh herbs of your choice, and serve warm.
8. Refrigerate any remaining broth.

BONE BROTH (BEEF)

This recipe uses beef bones instead of chicken bones. The method is mostly the same and the broth provides similar benefits.

Ingredients:

- 4 lb. beef bones – a mix of marrow bones, knuckle bones, short ribs, etc.
- 4 celery sticks, cut into 1 inch pieces

- 3 medium tomatoes, chopped
- 1 large onion, peeled and quartered
- 1 pound (2-3 medium) carrots, washed and cut into pieces
- 3-4 beets with leaves (leaves chopped, beets peeled and cut into pieces)
- 2 inch ginger piece, peeled and grated
- 3-4 cloves of garlic
- 1 gallon water
- Salt to taste
- Pepper to taste
- ½ cup cilantro
- ½ cup parsley
- 2 tbsp apple cider vinegar

Method

1. Add everything to a large pot. Bring to a boil.
2. Using a slotted spoon, remove any foam or scum that rises to the top and continue to skim the top until the broth is clear.
3. Reduce the heat and let it simmer for one hour. Remove any remaining fat or foam rising to the top.
4. Cover and simmer the broth for 18-24 hours.
5. Switch off the heat. Strain the broth into a large bowl using a mesh strainer.
6. Add salt to taste, add some chopped fresh herbs of your choice, and serve warm.

BONE BROTH (BEEF - SPICY)

This is a spicy version of the previous beef bone broth.

Basic Ingredients:

- 4 lb. beef bones – a mix of marrow bones, knuckle bones, short ribs, etc.
- 4 celery stalks, cut into 1 inch pieces
- 3 medium tomatoes, chopped
- 1 bell pepper, cut into pieces (any color)
- 1 large onion, peeled and quartered
- 1 pound (2-3 medium) carrots, washed and cut into pieces
- 1 gallon water
- 3 tbsp raw unfiltered apple cider vinegar
- Salt to taste (if you must or avoid salt)
- 2 tsp coconut oil

  Ingredients – spices and herbs
- 2 tsp turmeric powder
- 1 tsp cumin powder or cumin seeds
- 1 tsp coriander powder
- 1 tsp cayenne powder
- 2 tsp fenugreek seeds
- ½ cup parsley, chopped
- ½ cup cilantro, chopped
- ½ cup rosemary
- 3-4 garlic cloves, crushed
- 3-4 whole cloves
- 2 inch ginger root, peeled and grated
- 5-6 black peppercorns or ½ tsp pepper powder
- 1-2 bay leaves

Optional Ingredients

- 1-2 Jalapeño peppers split lengthwise

Method

1. In a medium pan, heat oil and crackle cumin seeds and fenugreek seeds. Add onion, crushed garlic, ginger, and jalapeño peppers.
2. Sauté for 2-3 minutes or until onion becomes translucent. Add all the remaining spices (cayenne, cumin, turmeric, coriander, cloves, bay leaves, pepper powder, etc.) and sauté for another 2-3 minutes so the spices are blended well and sufficiently roasted (make sure not to burn the spices).
3. Transfer the spice mix into a large pot (add some water to wash out any remaining spice mix from the pan and pour it into the large pot).
4. Add all beef bones and vegetables into pot along with the spices from step 3 and add water; bring to a boil.
5. Add vinegar. Lower the heat and simmer covered for 24-48 hours.
6. Once the bones and vegetables are cooked, strain the broth into a large bowl.
7. Add salt to taste, add some chopped fresh herbs of your choice, and serve warm.
8. Refrigerate any remaining broth.

BONE BROTH (LAMB - ROASTED)

Ingredients
- 3 lb. lamb bones with marrow
- 1 large onion, peeled and quartered
- 3 medium tomatoes, chopped
- 2 carrots, washed and cut into 1 inch long pieces
- 2 celery stalks, washed and cut into 1 inch pieces

- 1 inch ginger root, grated
- 3-4 garlic cloves, peeled and crushed
- 2-3 tbsp apple cider vinegar
- 2 tsp thyme
- ½ cup cilantro
- ¼ cup rosemary
- 1 gallon water
- Salt and pepper to taste

Method

1. Set oven to 350 degrees (176 degrees Celsius) and roast the lamb bones on a cooking sheet for about 45 minutes.
2. Add all roasted bones, vegetables, and other ingredients (except vinegar, salt, and pepper) into a large crock-pot. Add water and bring to a boil.
3. Add vinegar, lower the heat, and simmer covered for 24 hours.
4. Strain the broth into a large bowl. Add salt and pepper to taste. Add some fresh herbs of your choice (optional) and enjoy.
5. Refrigerate any remaining broth.

BONE BROTH (FISH)

Unlike other bone soups, fish bone soup takes less time to make and, in many cases, the bones will almost dissolve into the broth, especially if the bones are from small fish. Fishbone broth is extremely popular in some of the Asian countries and carries mostly the same benefits as other bone soups.

Ingredients

- 2 pounds of fish heads and bones, washed
- 3 medium tomatoes, chopped
- 1 inch ginger root, grated
- 3-4 garlic cloves, peeled and crushed
- 2-3 tsp apple cider vinegar
- ¼ cup cilantro, finely chopped
- 3 quarts water
- Salt and pepper to taste

Method

1. Put everything but salt and pepper in a pot and add water to cover the fish heads and bones. Bring to a boil and cook for 6 hours.
2. Strain the broth using a fine strainer.
3. Add salt and pepper to taste. Serve warm. The broth can be used in cooking other foods as well.

ENTRÉES AND OTHER DISHES

KALE CHIPS

Ingredients

- 1 bunch of red, green or Lacinato kale
- 2 tsp olive oil or garlic oil

Optional Ingredients

- A pinch of salt

Method

1. Preheat the oven to 350 degrees Fahrenheit (175 C.)
2. Use a knife to remove the thick stems from the leaves (the thick stems may be reused in soups or chili instead of discarding) and tear the leaves into small chip-sized pieces.
3. Put all the pieces in a mixing bowl, sprinkle with oil (olive or garlic oil) and salt (kale is a bit salty by itself so you can skip the salt depending on your taste) and mix well. Set it aside for 5 minutes before baking.
4. Bake for 10 minutes or until the kale pieces are crisp (be careful not to burn the chips).

SPINACH/RED CHARD STIR FRY

Basic Ingredients

- 4 cup chopped spinach or red chard
- ½ cup chopped onions
- 4-5 cloves crushed garlic
- 1 tsp turmeric powder
- 2 tsp coconut oil (or vegetable oil)
- Salt to taste
- 1 cup grated coconut

Optional Ingredients

- 2-3 dry red chilies
- 1 spring curry leaves
- ½ tsp mustard seeds
- 1 tsp cumin seeds

Method

1. Heat oil in a nonstick pan. Add optional mustard and cumin seeds and let it splutter.

2. Add onions, garlic, and optional curry leaves and red chilies and sauté for a couple of minutes until onions become translucent.
3. Add turmeric powder and sauté for a couple of minutes more.
4. Now add the chopped spinach or red chard and mix well. Cover and cook for 5-7 minutes, stirring occasionally to make sure no water remains.
5. Add grated coconut and salt, and mix.
6. Cook on low flame for 5 more minutes, stirring occasionally. Switch off the heat once spinach/chard is cooked and no water remains.

Serve as a side dish.

SALMON WITH GREEN MANGO

Basic Ingredients

- 2 lb. skinless salmon, cleaned and cut in 2 inch pieces
- 1-4 tsp chili powder (depending on your tolerance level)
- 1 tsp turmeric
- 1 tsp coriander powder
- ¼ tsp fenugreek powder or ½ tsp fenugreek seeds
- ¼ tsp black pepper powder
- ½ tsp mustard seeds
- 1 medium onion
- 2 tsp ginger root, grated
- 4-5 cloves garlic, crushed
- 2 cups washed and cut green mango (with skin or skin removed depending on your preference)

- 2 cups water (or as required)
- Salt to taste

Optional Ingredients

- 2 sprigs curry leaves
- 2-4 sliced green chilies or jalapeños, seeds removed

Method

1. To make masala paste, combine all the spice powders – chili, turmeric, coriander, fenugreek, and pepper powder – together in a bowl. Add 2 tsp or just enough water to make a thick paste and set aside.
2. Heat oil in a pan and splutter mustard seeds and fenugreek (if seeds are used instead of powder).
3. Add ginger, garlic, onion, and optional green chilies and curry leaves. Sauté until onion becomes translucent.
4. Add the masala paste and mix well on low flame. (Wet the masala to make sure it gets fried but not burnt.)
5. After a few minutes (once masala gets fried), add about 2 cups of water, mix and then add the cut mango pieces.
6. Cover it and bring it to a boil on medium heat. Now add individual fish pieces into the pan.
7. Mix gently, making sure the fish pieces are not broken up and that all the pieces are coated with the gravy.
8. Cover the pan and cook it for about 20 minutes or until fish is done and the gravy is thick. Switch off the flame

and keep it covered for 30 minutes for the fish to soak in the spices and mango flavor.

Serve with rice or bread.

Notes:

1. Paprika may be used instead of chili powder if you desire to make it less spicy.
2. Any other fish may be used instead of salmon.
3. Instead of mango, tamarind or *Garcinia cambogia* (the scientific name for black tamarind available in Asian stores) may be used.
4. Green chilies or jalapeños add more heat to the fish curry. Use it depending on your taste.

OVEN-BAKED SALMON

Ingredients

- 4 salmon fillets (5-6 ounces each)
- 2 teaspoons olive oil
- 1 teaspoon turmeric powder
- ½ -1 teaspoon black pepper powder
- ¼ cup chopped cilantro
- ¼ parsley flakes
- 2 garlic cloves, finely chopped
- 2 teaspoons lemon juice
- ½ -1 teaspoon salt (or to taste)

Optional Ingredients

- ½ inch ginger root, grated

Method

1. Place the salmon fillets skin down on a well-greased (olive oil or butter) glass baking dish (sufficiently large to hold the 4 pieces).
2. Put the other ingredients – garlic, ginger, turmeric, black pepper, lemon juice, salt, and olive oil – in a small bowl and mix well.
3. Coat the spice, oil and lemon mixture on each of the fillets.
4. Now cover the fillets with cilantro and parsley by sprinkling the herbs on top.
5. Bake for 18-20 minutes at 375 degrees Fahrenheit.

BROCCOLI STIR FRY

Basic Ingredients

- 2 lb. broccoli florets washed
- 2 tsp coconut oil (olive oil or vegetable oil can be used instead)
- 1 tsp turmeric powder
- 1 medium onion, sliced
- ¼ tsp black pepper powder
- Salt to taste

Optional Ingredients

- 1 Jalapeño pepper, sliced into thin pieces (seeds out)
- 1 tsp mustard seeds
- ½ cup cilantro
- ½ cup parsley
- ½ tsp fresh lemon juice

Method

6. Heat oil in a medium nonstick pan; crackle optional mustard seeds in oil.
7. Add onion and optional jalapeño pepper. Stir until golden.
8. Add turmeric and black pepper, stir for one minute and then add broccoli florets and mix well until the broccoli is coated with the turmeric.
9. Cover the pan with a lid and cook for 5-10 minutes on low-medium heat stirring occasionally. Once cooked, switch off heat; add the optional cilantro, and parsley. Add salt to taste. Add optional lemon juice.

Mix well and serve hot. Usually, there is no need to add water. At low heat, the moisture in the broccoli will help it to cook well.

BELL PEPPER AND CHICKEN STIR FRY

Basic Ingredients

- 1 bell pepper, washed and cut into thin slices (any color)
- 2 tsp coconut oil (olive oil or vegetable oil can be used instead)
- 1 lb. boneless chicken breast, cut into thin strips
- 1 tsp turmeric powder
- 1 tsp black pepper powder
- 1 tsp coriander powder
- 1 medium onion, sliced
- ½ inch piece ginger root, thinly sliced
- Salt to taste
- 1-2 medium tomatoes, sliced
- 3 cloves garlic, crushed

Optional Ingredients

- 1 Jalapeño pepper, sliced into thin pieces
- ¼ cup cilantro, chopped

Method

1. Sprinkle ½ teaspoons of turmeric powder, pepper powder, and salt on the washed and cut chicken. Mix well, and set aside for 10 minutes.
2. In a pan, heat oil, and add onion, crushed garlic, ginger, and optional Jalapeño. Sauté until onion becomes translucent.
3. Add the rest of the turmeric powder, coriander powder, and pepper powder and mix well.
4. Add tomatoes and mix.
5. Now add the bell pepper and chicken and mix well.
6. Cover and cook for 10 minutes on medium heat or until chicken and peppers are cooked. Stir occasionally.
7. Switch off the heat, and add optional cilantro. Add more salt if required, depending on your taste.

Serve with rice or bread.

COCONUT CURRY CHICKEN

Basic Ingredients

- 1-1/2 pounds chicken breast, cut into small (1 inch) pieces
- 2-4 teaspoons curry powder, depending on your tolerance to the spice

- 1 tsp turmeric
- 1 medium onion, chopped
- 2-3 tsp coconut oil (olive oil or vegetable oil can be used instead)
- ½ tsp pepper powder
- 2 medium potatoes, peeled and cut into 1 inch cubes
- 3-4 cloves garlic, crushed
- ½ inch cube ginger root, peeled and sliced
- 1 can (14 oz.) coconut milk
- ¼ cup mint leaves or cilantro
- Salt to taste
- ½ -1 can chicken broth (depending on the amount of gravy desired)

Optional Ingredients

- 1 cup carrots, sliced
- 2 medium tomatoes, chopped

Method

1. Sprinkle 1 tsp curry powder, ½ tsp turmeric and ¼ tsp salt, on cut chicken. Mix well and set it aside for 10 minutes.
2. In a separate pan, heat oil, sauté onion, garlic, and ginger until onion becomes translucent.
3. Add remaining curry powder, turmeric, and pepper powder. Mix for 1-2 minutes.
4. Add chicken, potatoes, and optional tomatoes and carrots. Mix well 1-2 minutes until the chicken and potatoes are coated with the gravy.
5. Add chicken broth and bring it to a boil. Stir well.

6. Reduce heat to low medium, cover the pan and cook for 10-12 minutes or until chicken, potatoes and carrots are well mixed, the chicken loses its pink color, and potatoes and carrots are about half cooked.

7. Add coconut milk and cover. Simmer on low heat for another 20 minutes or until chicken, potatoes and carrots are cooked well and soft.

8. Add mint leaves/cilantro and stir. Add salt to taste. Switch off the heat and keep it covered for 1-2 minutes before serving.

Serve with rice or bread.

CAULIFLOWER AND POTATO

Basic Ingredients

- 2 medium potatoes, peeled and cut into 1 inch cubes
- ½ head cauliflower washed and cut into small pieces (same size as potatoes)
- 2 tsp coconut oil (olive oil or vegetable oil can be used instead)
- ½ tsp black pepper powder
- 1 medium onion, sliced
- 1 tsp turmeric
- 1-2 medium tomatoes, chopped
- Salt to taste
- ¼ cup cilantro, chopped
- ½ cup vegetable broth

Optional Ingredients
- ½ tsp cumin seeds

- 1-2 Jalapeños, sliced (seeds removed if desired)
- 2-3 cloves of garlic, crushed
- ½ inch ginger, chopped into fine pieces
- ½-1 tsp curry powder

Method

1. Heat oil in a medium nonstick pan, and crackle optional cumin seeds.
2. Add onion, and optional garlic, ginger, and Jalapeños. Stir until onion becomes translucent.
3. Add turmeric, black pepper, and optional curry powder, and stir for 1-2 minutes.
4. Add chopped tomatoes, potatoes and cauliflower, mix well and then add vegetable broth.
5. Bring to a boil, stirring intermittently.
6. Cover and simmer for 10-15 minutes or until the potatoes and cauliflower are cooked.
7. Switch off heat; add the cilantro and salt.

Mix well and serve hot as a side dish with rice or bread.

Recipe Notes:

1. There are many optional ingredients listed, one could use all of them or pick and choose based on your taste.
2. The Jalapeños vary in their heat level. If you choose to use them, you can take the seeds out to reduce the heat. This note applies to all the recipes in this book.

TOMATO RICE

This is a good way to color your rice and include turmeric, ginger and garlic as part of the diet.

Basic Ingredients

- 2 cups basmati rice
- 1 tsp turmeric powder
- 2 tsp coconut oil (olive oil or vegetable oil can be used instead)
- 1 pinch black pepper powder
- 3 medium tomatoes, chopped
- 1 medium onion, chopped
- Salt to taste
- ¼ cup cilantro, chopped

Optional Ingredients

- ½ tsp mustard seeds
- ½ cumin seeds
- 1-2 Jalapeños, sliced
- 3 cloves garlic, crushed
- ½ inch piece ginger root, thinly sliced

Method

1. Cook the rice in a rice cooker or on the stovetop, then drain (if needed) and set aside.
2. In a medium pan (big enough to mix rice), heat oil, and crackle optional mustard and cumin seeds.
3. Add onion, and optional garlic, ginger, and Jalapeños; sauté until the onion is golden brown.
4. Add turmeric and pepper and mix. Now add the tomatoes; mix.

5. Cover and cook for 10 minutes on medium heat or until tomatoes are cooked well.
6. Add the cooked rice, mix it well, and add salt to taste.
7. Add chopped cilantro and serve.

BEEF/CHICKEN PEPPER FRY

Ingredients

- 2 lbs. boneless chicken breast/beef, cut into 1 inch cubes/strips
- 2 tsp coconut oil (olive oil or vegetable oil can be used instead)
- ½ tsp turmeric powder
- 1-2 tsp black pepper powder
- 2 tsp coriander powder
- 2 large onions, sliced
- 2 inches piece ginger root, thinly sliced
- Salt
- 2-3 medium tomatoes, sliced
- 4-6 cloves garlic, crushed

Optional Ingredients

- 1 cup cilantro

Method

1. Heat oil in a medium nonstick pan; add onions, garlic, and ginger. Stir until golden.
2. Add coriander powder, pepper powder, and turmeric. Stir for 2-3 minutes.
3. Add tomatoes and mix well.

4. Add chicken and mix so that chicken is coated well with spices and onions.
5. Cover and simmer for 20-25 minutes or until the chicken is cooked, stirring occasionally so the chicken or the gravy does not stick to the pan.
6. Garnish with optional cilantro. Serve with rice or naan (Indian bread).

KALE AND CHICKEN FRY

This is something I tried recently and found good. The simplest way to make this is to make chicken with spices following any one of the recipes above, make kale chips and just crumble the chips into the chicken and mix well.

Ingredients

- 2 lbs. boneless chicken breast/beef, cut into 1 inch cubes/strips
- 2 tsp coconut oil (olive oil or vegetable oil can be used instead)
- ½ tsp turmeric powder
- 1-2 tsp black pepper powder
- 2 tsp coriander powder
- 2 large onions, sliced
- 2 inch piece ginger root, thinly sliced
- Salt to taste
- 2-3 medium tomatoes, sliced
- 4-6 cloves garlic, crushed
- 2 cups green or red kale, washed and cut/tore into 1-2 inch pieces (to make kale chips)

Optional Ingredients

- 1 cup cilantro

Method

1. Heat oil in a medium nonstick pan; add onions, garlic, and ginger. Stir until golden.
2. Add coriander powder, pepper powder, and turmeric, stir for one minute, and then add tomatoes and mix well.
3. Add chicken and mix so that chicken is coated well with spices and onions.
4. Cover and simmer for 20-25 minutes or until the chicken is cooked, stirring occasionally so the chicken or the gravy does not stick to the pan.
5. Meanwhile, at the same time, spread the kale pieces on a cookie sheet and put in the oven at 350 degrees for 10 minutes or until the kale pieces become chips and can easily crumble.
6. Once the chicken is cooked, take the kale chips and crumble using your hand and spread on top of the chicken fry.
7. Mix well and cover it for 1 minute. Garnish with cilantro. Serve with rice or naan (Indian bread).

CHAPTER 6. SUMMARY

I hope this book provides you with some understanding of the Alzheimer's factors to avoid as well as insight into the various methods of preventing, delaying the onset or reversing Alzheimer's. The use of spices and herbs, with their medicinal properties, helps transform any meal into a healthy and disease-fighting meal. While a lot of focus in this book is on prevention through food, other prevention methods are as important. Here is my list of the top 6 things to prevent, delay the onset of, and slow down the progression of Alzheimer's.

1. Be a lifelong learner, be active mentally

- Learn something new every day, every week, every month. Look back at the end of the day and think about what you learned that day. As part of your New Year's resolutions, plan to learn one new skill a year. It could be:

    ◦ Learn a musical instrument.

    ◦ Learn a new language.

    ◦ Learn a new hobby such as knitting or crocheting.

    ◦ Learning chess, checkers or any strategy game.

- Learn a new subject or topic related to your work.

- Keep mentally active.

  - Play games such as sudoku, scrabble, ken-ken, crossword puzzles, or cards.

  - Play brain teasers and trivia games

  - Play games on Lumosity or other brain training apps.

  - Keep a diary or journal to write down daily experiences of "who, what, where, when, and why". The process of writing things down helps to improve memory. Describe everything as vividly as possible. Visualize the events before writing them down.

  - Practice memorization. Take it up as a hobby. Try to remember names, numbers (phone number, credit card number), and facts (state names, country names, capitals). Visualize and associate names with people and objects.

2. **Be aware and conscious about what you eat or drink.**

- Eat more of the brain foods identified in this book.

- Eat more colorful vegetables and fruits.

- Limit/avoid processed foods.

- Limit/avoid sodas of any kind.

- Eat more vegan and organic protein.

- Limit sugar intake.

- Limit alcohol consumption.

- Limit salt. Be aware many off the shelf and processed foods have too much sodium.

- Eat freshly prepared foods whenever possible. Cook at home more often. It makes not only short term and long term economic sense but is healthful as well.

- Use spices and herbs – especially turmeric, garlic, and ginger (and others such as cinnamon, chili powder, etc.) – in the preparation of foods that help fight inflammation and neutralize free radicals.

- Recently, it has been reported that some common prescription medications (anticholinergic drugs) can increase the risk of dementia as much as 50%. Consult your physician if you are on anticholinergic prescription drugs.

3. **Be physically active.**

- Be aware of how much time you exercise, and how much time you sit on the sofa or sit at the workplace.

- Exercise at least 30 minutes a day. Pick up a physical activity that you enjoy. Enlist other people so you can exercise in groups or teams where you can feed off each other and maintain the motivation.

- Hit the gym or pick up running, walking, or a team game such as tennis, volleyball, basketball, etc.

- Join senior leagues for sports and physical activities.

- Practice yoga or tai chi, which provide many benefits including:

  ○ improved balance and coordination that help in your old age; especially your balance is impacted by Alzheimer's

  ○ stress reduction again, they help in reducing stress on the brain

4. Be aware of your family's medical history.

- While your DNA/genetics is something one cannot change, being aware of family history helps one to take preventive and cautionary steps that can certainly either completely prevent or reduce the risk of getting Alzheimer's.

- While only 5% of all Alzheimer's patients are due to genetic factors, if you know if your close relatives had Alzheimer's, you are at increased risk. This knowledge gives you the power to change your lifestyle and practice prevention at an early age.

5. Improve the quality of sleep.

- Sleep time is used by the brain for memory formation. The whole body uses sleep as a restorative process to recover from all the work the body did during the hours awake.

- Sleep helps to flush out toxins from the brain and prevent the formation of beta-amyloid plaques in the brain that increases the risk for Alzheimer's.

6. Protect your heart and head.

- Cardio-vascular problems can increase the risk of Alzheimer's.
- Follow a diet and exercise regimen to improve cardiovascular health.
- Protect your head from injury by wearing a helmet when appropriate and fall-proofing your home.

I wish you all the best in your journey towards Alzheimer's free future!

DISCLAIMER

This book details the author's personal experiences in using Indian spices and information contained in the public domain, as well as the author's opinion. The author is not licensed as a doctor, nutritionist or chef. The author is providing this book and its contents on an "as is" basis and makes no representations or warranties of any kind with respect to this book or its contents. The author disclaims all such representations and warranties, including for example warranties of merchantability and educational or medical advice for a particular purpose. In addition, the author does not represent or warrant that the information accessible via this book is accurate, complete or current. The statements made about products and services have not been evaluated by the US FDA or any equivalent organization in other countries.

The author will not be liable for damages arising out of or in connection with the use of this book or the information contained within. This is a comprehensive limitation of liability that applies to all damages of any kind, including (without limitation) compensatory; direct, indirect or consequential damages; loss of data, income or profit; loss of or damage to property and claims of third parties. It is understood that this book is not intended as a substitute for consultation with a licensed medical or a culinary professional. Before starting any lifestyle changes, it is recommended that you consult a licensed professional to ensure that you are doing what's best for your situation. The use of this book implies your acceptance of this disclaimer.

Thank You

If you enjoyed this book or found it useful I would greatly appreciate if you could post a short review on Amazon. I read all the reviews and your feedback will help me to make this book even better. For your convenience, please click the following link to take you directly to Amazon where you can post the review:

https://www.amazon.com/dp/B077LKRTHD

Appendix I. Sources And References

This book was written based on the author's personal experience with super foods and spices as well as information from a wide range of sources. Some of the key sources are outlined below, in case the reader would like to read more details about Alzheimer's and its prevention.

15 Brain Foods That Boost Memory

https://draxe.com/15-brain-foods-to-boost-focus-and-memory/

Alzheimer's death rate by country

HTTP://WWW.WORLDLIFEEXPECTANCY.COM/CAUSE-OF-DEATH/ALZHEIMERS-DEMENTIA/BY-COUNTRY/

2017 Alzheimer's Facts and figures

HTTPS://WWW.ALZ.ORG/DOCUMENTS_CUSTOM/2017-FACTS-AND-FIGURES.PDF

Optimizing diagnosis and management in mild-to-moderate Alzheimer's disease

HTTPS://WWW.NCBI.NLM.NIH.GOV/PMC/ARTICLES/PMC343
7664/

Health benefits of Eggs

https://www.huffingtonpost.com/2013/03/30/health-benefits-of-eggs-yolks_n_2966554.html

Leafy green vegetables and brain health

https://consumer.healthday.com/senior-citizen-information-31/misc-aging-news-10/lots-of-leafy-greens-might-shield-aging-brains-study-finds-697909.html

Walnuts and memory

https://www.huffingtonpost.com/2015/01/22/walnuts-boost-memory-study_n_6525316.html

6 brain foods good for the mind

http://www.telegraph.co.uk/news/science/science-news/11364896/Brain-food-6-snacks-that-are-good-for-the-mind.html

Eat smart for a healthier brain

https://www.webmd.com/diet/features/eat-smart-healthier-brain#1

Omega-3 fatty acids and their role in central nervous system

https://www.ncbi.nlm.nih.gov/pubmed/26795198

Vitamin B12 and Omega-3 effects on brain function

https://www.ncbi.nlm.nih.gov/pubmed/26809263

Fish consumption and cognitive decline with age

https://www.ncbi.nlm.nih.gov/pubmed/16216930

Neuro-protective effects of berries on neurodegenerative diseases

https://www.ncbi.nlm.nih.gov/pmc/articles/PMC4192974/

Blueberries improve memory in older adults

https://www.ncbi.nlm.nih.gov/pmc/articles/PMC2850944/

Neuroprotective properties of turmeric

http://www.eurekaselect.com/76132

http://www.nature.com/articles/srep38846

http://articles.mercola.com/sites/articles/archive/2013/07/08/
-vs-drugs-for-parkinsons.aspx

http://www.sciencedirect.com/science/article/pii/S13572725
08002550

Anti-inflammatory properties of turmeric

https://www.ncbi.nlm.nih.gov/pubmed/19594223

https://www.ncbi.nlm.nih.gov/pubmed/12676044

Broccoli benefits

https://www.ncbi.nlm.nih.gov/pmc/articles/PMC3725709/

Chocolate intake associated with better cognitive function

https://www.ncbi.nlm.nih.gov/pubmed/26873453

Nuts and cognitive function

https://www.ncbi.nlm.nih.gov/pmc/articles/PMC4105147/

Neurological mechanisms of green tea in Alzheimer's and
Parkinson's

https://www.ncbi.nlm.nih.gov/pubmed/15350981

10 foods to boost your brain power

https://www.bbcgoodfood.com/howto/guide/10-foods-boost-your-brainpower

Oral Health and Alzheimer's Risk

https://www.beingpatient.com/oral-care-dementia-gum-disease/

Some very good TED Talks on Alzheimer's

https://www.ted.com/talks/lisa_genova_what_you_can_do_to_prevent_alzheimer_s

https://www.ted.com/talks/alanna_shaikh_how_i_m_preparing_to_get_alzheimer_s

PREVIEW OF OTHER BOOKS IN THIS SERIES

ESSENTIAL SPICES AND HERBS: TURMERIC

Turmeric is truly a wonder spice. It has anti-inflammatory, anti-oxidant, anti-cancer, and anti-bacterial properties. Find out the amazing benefits of turmeric. Includes many recipes for incorporating turmeric in your daily life.

Turmeric is a spice known to man for thousands of years and has been used for cooking, food preservation, and as a natural remedy for common ailments. This book explains:

- Many health benefits of turmeric including fighting cancer, inflammation, and pain.
- Turmeric as beauty treatments - turmeric masks
- Recipes for teas, smoothies and dishes
- References and links to a number of research studies on the effectiveness of turmeric

Essential Spices and Herbs: Turmeric is a quick read and offers a lot of concise information. A great tool to have in your alternative therapies and healthy lifestyle toolbox!

PREVENTING CANCER

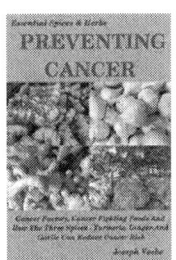 World Health Organization (WHO) estimates more than half of all cancer incidents are preventable.

Cancer is one of the most fearsome diseases to strike mankind. There has been much research into both conventional and alternative therapies for different kinds of cancers. Different cancers require different treatment options and offer a different prognosis. While there has been significant progress in recent times in cancer research towards a cure, there are none available currently. However, more than half of all cancers are likely preventable through modifications in lifestyle and diet.

Preventing Cancer offers a quick insight into cancer-causing factors, foods that fight cancer, and how the three spices, turmeric, ginger and garlic, can not only spice up your food but potentially make all your food into cancer fighting meals. While there are many other herbs and spices that help fight cancer, these three spices work together and complementarily. In addition, the medicinal value of these spices has been proven over thousands of years of use. The book includes:

- Cancer-causing factors and how to avoid them
- Top 12 cancer-fighting foods, the cancers they fight and how to incorporate them into your diet
- Cancer-fighting properties of turmeric, ginger and garlic

- Over 30 recipes including teas, smoothies and other dishes that incorporate these spices
- References and links to many research studies on the effectiveness of these spices.

PREVENTING ALZHEIMER'S

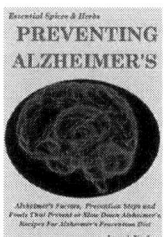Approximately 50 million people suffer from Alzheimer's worldwide. In the U.S. alone, 5.5 million people have Alzheimer's – about 10 percent of the worldwide Alzheimer's population.

Alzheimer's disease is a progressive brain disorder that damages and eventually destroys brain cells, leading to memory loss, changes in thinking, and other brain functions. While the rate of progressive decline in brain function is slow at the onset, it gets worse with time and age. Brain function decline accelerates, and brain cells eventually die over time. While there has been significant research done to find a cure, currently there is no cure available.

Alzheimer's incidence rate in the U.S. and other western countries is significantly higher than that of the countries in the developing world. Factors such as lifestyle, diet, physical and mental activity, and social engagement play a part in the development and progression of Alzheimer's

In most cases, if you are above the age of 50, plaques and tangles associated with Alzheimer's may have already started forming in your brain. At the age of 65, you have a 10% chance of Alzheimer's and at age 80, the chances are about 50%.

With lifestyle changes, proper diet and exercise (of the mind and body), Alzheimer's is preventable.

In recent times, Alzheimer's is beginning to reach epidemic proportions. The cost of Alzheimer's to the US economy is expected to cross a trillion dollars in 10 years. It is a serious health care issue in many of the western countries as the population age and the life expectancy increase.

At this time, our understanding of what causes Alzheimer's and the ways to treat it is at its infancy. However, we know the factors that affect Alzheimer's and we can use that knowledge to prevent, delay the onset or at least slow down the rate of progression of the disease.

While this book does not present all the answers, it is an attempt to examines the factors affecting Alzheimer's and how to reduce the risk of developing Alzheimer's. A combination of diet and both mental and physical exercise is believed to help in prevention or reducing risk. The book includes:

Discussion on factors in Alzheimer's development

The list of foods that help protect the brain and boost brain health is included in the book:

Over 30 recipes including teas, smoothies, broths, and other dishes that incorporate brain-boosting foods:

References and links to several research studies on Alzheimer's and brain foods.

ALL NATURAL WELLNESS DRINKS

It contains 35 recipes for wellness drinks that include teas, smoothies, soups, and vegan & bone broths. The recipes in this book are unique and combine superfoods, medicinal spices, and herbs. These drinks are anti-cancer, anti-diabetic, ant-aging, heart healthy, anti-inflammatory, and anti-oxidant as well as promote weight loss.

By infusing nature-based nutrients (super fruits and vegetables, spices, and herbs) into drink recipes, we get some amazing wellness drinks that not only replace water loss but nourish the body with vitamins, essential metals, anti-oxidants, and many other nutrients. These drinks may be further enhanced by incorporating spices and herbs along with other superfoods. These drinks not only help heal the body but also enhance the immune system to help prevent many forms of diseases. These drinks may also help rejuvenate the body and delay the aging process. The book also includes suggested wellness drinks for common ailments.

ESSENTIAL SPICES AND HERBS: GINGER

Ginger is a spice known to man for thousands of years and has been used for cooking and as a natural remedy for common ailments. Recent studies have shown that ginger has anti-cancer, anti-inflammatory, and anti-oxidant properties. Ginger helps in reducing muscle pain and is an excellent remedy for nausea. Ginger promotes a healthy digestive system. The book details:

- Many health benefits of ginger including fighting cancer, inflammation, pain and nausea
- Remedies using ginger
- Recipes for teas, smoothies, and other dishes
- References and links to a number of research studies on the effectiveness of ginger

ESSENTIAL SPICES AND HERBS: GARLIC

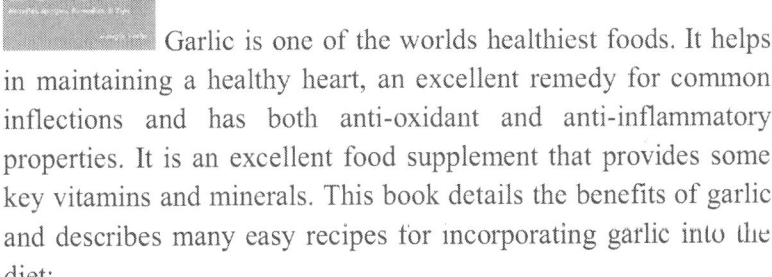 Garlic is one of the worlds healthiest foods. It helps in maintaining a healthy heart, an excellent remedy for common inflections and has both anti-oxidant and anti-inflammatory properties. It is an excellent food supplement that provides some key vitamins and minerals. This book details the benefits of garlic and describes many easy recipes for incorporating garlic into the diet:

- Many health benefits of garlic including fighting cancer, inflammation, heart health and more
- Remedies using garlic
- Recipes for teas, smoothies, and other dishes
- References and links to a number of research studies on the effectiveness of garlic

ESSENTIAL SPICES AND HERBS: CINNAMON

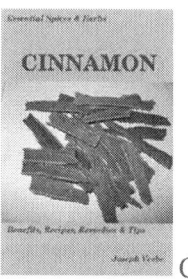 Cinnamon is an essential spice. It has Anti-diabetic, anti-inflammatory, anti-oxidant, anti-cancer and anti-infections and neuroprotective properties. Cinnamon is a spice known to man for thousands of years and has been used for food preservation, baking, cooking, and as a natural remedy for common ailments. Recent studies have shown that cinnamon has important medicinal properties. This book explains:

- Many health benefits of cinnamon including anti-diabetic, neuroprotective and others.
- Recipes for teas, smoothies, and other dishes
- References and links to a number of research studies on the effectiveness of cinnamon

ANTI-CANCER CURRIES

It is estimated that more than 50% of the cancer incidents are preventable by changing lifestyles, controlling or avoiding cancer-causing factors, or simply eating healthy. There are several foods that are known to have anti-cancer properties either directly or indirectly. Some of these have properties that inhibit cancer cell growth while others have antioxidant and anti-inflammatory properties that contribute to overall health. However, many spices and herbs have direct anti-cancer properties and when one uses anti-cancer spices and herbs in cooking fresh food, there is an immense benefit to be gained. Curry dishes are cooked using many spices that have anti-oxidant, anti-inflammatory, and anti-cancer properties.

This book contains 30 curry recipes that use healthy and anti-cancer ingredients. These recipes are simple and take an average of 20-30 minutes to prepare.

BEGINNERS GUIDE TO COOKING WITH SPICES

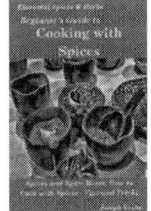 Have you ever wondered how to cook with spices? Learn about the many benefits of spices and how to cook with them!

Find out how to start using spices as seasoning and healthy foods. Includes sample recipes,

Beginner's guide to cooking with spices is an introductory book that explains the history, various uses, and their medicinal properties and health benefits. The book details how they may be easily incorporated in everyday cooking. The book will cover the following:

- Health benefits of spices and herbs
- Spice mixes from around the world and their uses
- Tips for cooking with Spices
- Cooking Vegan with Spices
- Cooking Meat and Fish with spices
- Spiced Rice Dishes
- Spicy Soups and Broths

EASY INDIAN INSTANT POT COOKBOOK

Instant Pot or Electric Pressure Cooker is the most important cooking device in my kitchen. It saves me time, energy, and helps me prepare hassle-free Indian meals all the time.

The Easy Indian Instant Pot Meals contains includes:
- Recipes for 50 Indian dishes
- Tips for cooking with Instant Pot or any electric pressure cooker
- General tips for cooking with spices

FIGHTING THE VIRUS: HOW TO BOOST YOUR BODY'S IMMUNE RESPONSE AND FIGHT VIRUS NATURALLY

What can we do to improve our health and immune response so that our bodies are less prone to viral or bacterial infections? How can we enable our body for a speedy recovery in case of getting such infections?

The answer lies in lifestyle changes that include better hygiene practices, exercise, sleep, and a better diet to keep our body in optimum health. This book is focused on understanding the body's immune system, factors that improve the body's immune response and some natural remedies and recipes. The book contains:
•Overview of the human immune system

•Factors affecting immune response
•Natural substances that fight viral, fungal and bacterial infections
•Recipes that may improve immunity and help speedy recovery
•Supplements that may help improve the immune system
•Scientific studies and references

EASY SPICY EGGS: ALL NATURAL EASY AND SPICY EGG RECIPES

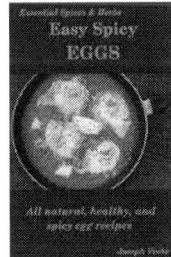 Recipes in this book are not a collection of authentic dishes, but a spicy version of chicken recipes that are easy to make and 100% healthy and flavorful. Ingredients used are mostly natural without any preserved or processed foods.

Most of these recipes include tips and tricks to vary and adapt to your taste of spice level or make with some of the ingredients you like other than the prescribed ingredients in the recipes.

There are about 30 recipes in the book with ideas to make another 30 or even more with the suggestions and notes included with many of the recipes. Cooking does not have to be prescriptive but can be creative. I invite you to try your own variations and apply your creativity to cook dishes that are truly your own.

FOOD FOR THE BRAIN

Nature provides for foods that nourish both the body and the brain. Most often the focus of the diet is physical nourishment, - muscle building, weight loss, energy, athletic performance, and many others. Similar to foods that help the body, there are many foods that help the brain, improve memory and help slow down the aging process. While it is normal to have your physical and mental abilities somewhat slow down with age, diseases such as Alzheimer's, and Parkinson's impact these declines even more. Brain function decline accelerates, and more and more brain cells eventually die over time.

With regular exercises, strength training, practicing martial arts and other physical activities can arrest the physical decline. This book's primary focus is on managing decline in mental and brain function through diet and contains the following:
Characteristics of foods that helps in keeping your brain healthy and young. Brain healthy foods including meats, fruits, vegetables, spices, herbs, and seafood. Supplements to improve memory, cognition and support brain health
Mediterranean diet recipe ideas
DASH diet recipe ideas
Asian diet recipe ideas
Brain boosting supplements and recommendations products and dosage
References

Printed in Great Britain
by Amazon